Comments and Reviews about Quick & Healthy…

Recommended in *O, The Oprah Magazine*.

"Here's one cookbook that lives up to its name…." —*Cooking Light Magazine*

"Well organized, well-thought-out, takes into account how busy most of us really are…. This could become a kitchen standby for busy cooks…." —*Miami Herald*

"My patients love these user-friendly books. It is great for diabetics and people with heart disease and high cholesterol levels. What I love is the practical weight loss tips, time saving ideas, and practical nutrition guidelines. I highly recommend this cookbook for every one who wants to cook healthy and has no time to cook!" —**Julie Conner, RD, MPH, PhD, President of Healthy Weighs**

"A lifesaver for real-world cooks … with a wealth of dietary hints and shortcuts." —*BookPage*

"My favorite cookbooks, focused on healthy, quick recipes, include the *Quick & Healthy* series by Brenda J. Ponichtera." —**David L. Katz, MD, director of Yale-Griffin Prevention Research Center and medical consultant for *ABC News***

"Superbly organized. Showcases delicious, 'heart healthy,' diabetes appropriate, weight control friendly recipes." —*Midwest Book Review*

"This health-conscious cookbook is the best I have seen—providing simple, easy-to-read, accurate information that focuses on today's issues…. Brenda Ponichtera is an expert at translating good, sound scientific facts into the practical." —**Barbara Craven, PhD, RD, consumer educator for Whole Foods Markets and U.S. federal agencies**

"Many new cookbooks include the word 'healthy' in the title, but if you're looking for information and recipes that are also quick and useful, this cookbook will be a good investment. These are not gourmet dishes with a long list of hard-to-find ingredients." —*The Oregonian*

"A fantastic find for busy people who want to cook at home and prepare meals that will promote a healthier lifestyle. This book is packed with practical tips on shopping, motivating reminders, sound and up-to-date nutrition information, and quick, easy, and delicious recipes. This rare treasure is especially helpful for someone who wants to learn how to cook healthy meals or wants variety in their menus!" —**Monica A. Cengia, MSEd, RD, CDE, Diabetes Educator and Nutrition Consultant**

"I'm thrilled to finally have a cookbook that I can wholeheartedly recommend to all my patients…." —**Kathy K. Isold, MS, RD, CDE, The Comprehensive Weight Control Center, New York**

"One way to eat healthier: modify fat-laden recipes. *Quick & Healthy* is one of ten that the National Center for Nutrition and Dietetics suggest you consider." —*USA Today*

"A great book to recommend to clients, family, and friends." —**Kathryn Miller, MS, RD, LD, Staff Nutritionist, Cooper Clinic, Dallas, Texas**

"Not only are the recipes appealing, the book is rich in imaginative and creative tips for 'quick and healthy' shopping, cooking, and menu ideas…. It's a book that dietitians will feel confident in recommending as well as giving for a gift." —**Marion J. Franz, RD, MS, CDE, International Diabetes Center, Minneapolis, Minnesota**

"I can say with confidence, *Quick & Healthy* should be on every cookbook shelf."
—Carol M. Meerschaert, RD, LDN

"…contains easy-to-follow, healthful recipes that your family will actually eat." —*California Health*

"The recipes are designed to be low in fat and cholesterol, yet high in taste. This practical 'how-to' guide includes menus, ideas for no-cook meals, weight control suggestions, food products worth selecting … and even the shopping list! I recommend that you buy this book." —Nancy Clark, MS, RD, Sports Nutritionist and author of *Nancy Clark's Sports Nutrition Guidebook*

"At last. Practical tips for controlling fat and cholesterol, along with quick, healthy recipes that taste great. Highly recommended." —John P. Foreyt, PhD, Director, Nutrition Research Clinic, Houston, Texas

"Resolutions to eat healthier are easy to do using *Quick & Healthy*. The recipes work, and what's more, they taste like you've been slaving over them for hours." —*The Single Parent*

"Just what people are looking for—a user friendly book about a lower fat, higher complex carbohydrate eating style." —Sonja L. Conner, MS, RD, Research Associate Professor, Oregon Health Sciences University and co-author of *The New American Diet*

"*Quick & Healthy* is not just another cookbook. The Time Saving Ideas, Quick Meals and Grocery Lists make the book more like a kitchen almanac…. A must-have for today's busy cooks!" —Peggy Paul, RD, LD, Director, Oregon Dairy Council

"Brenda's a mom, too, and knows what it takes to try to make all the eaters in the family happy." —*Farmers Advance*

"…targets all of us who claim we do not have time to eat healthfully. A worthwhile addition to any 'eat and run' kitchen." —*Lipid Clinic News*

"After a long day at work, no one wants to spend hours in the kitchen cooking. Author, educator, and registered dietitian Brenda Ponichtera understands that and she planned her book accordingly. Her book offers great timesaving tips, practical nutrition information, easy-to-prepare recipes, and even a master grocery list. More than a traditional cookbook, *Quick & Healthy* is an anthology of ideas for healthy living." —*Focus on Books*

"Easy-to-fix recipes for low-fat meals." —*The Columbian*

"I find it to be more than just a cookbook. It is also a guide to nutrition, and provides lessons about food and dieting throughout the book. I would definitely recommend it to someone who is looking for a healthier way to eat." —Pamela La Gioia, President, *Your Life! Magazine*

"These quick-fix meals don't skimp on health." —*The Register-Guard*

"A Must-Have for Improving Your Diet. I use this book plus Ponichtera's other *Quick & Healthy* books with patients and in my own home. I work in the food and nutrition profession where we focus on getting folks to eat better and healthier. Telling them how is part of the battle, and showing them how with delicious, easy and quick recipes is the other component. I highly recommend this book!" —D. Milton Stokes, RD, Clinical Nutrition Manager, North General Hospital, New York

"This book is a must have." —Tracy Farnsworth, roundtablereviews.com

"Excellent cookbook addressing low fat with balanced health maintenance and prevention focus. Uses common ingredients! A must buy!" —Dianne Smith, RN, Cardiopulmonary and Vascular Rehabilitation, Bellin Health

Quick

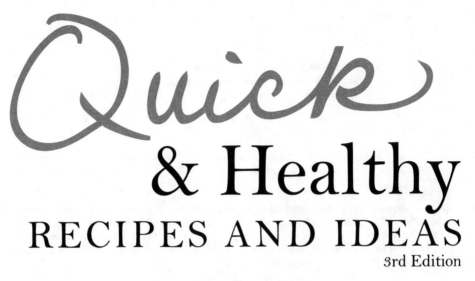

& Healthy

RECIPES AND IDEAS

3rd Edition

For people who say
they don't have time to cook healthy meals

Brenda J. Ponichtera
REGISTERED DIETITIAN

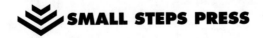 **SMALL STEPS PRESS**

Director, Book Publishing, Robert Anthony; *Managing Editor, Book Publishing,* Abe Ogden; *Production Manager,* Melissa Sprott; *Cover Design,* Vis-a-Vis Creative; *Illustrations,* Lisa Becharas, Janice Staver; *Printer,* United Graphics, Inc.

Printed in the United States of America

1 3 5 7 9 10 8 6 4 2

Small Steps Press is an imprint of the American Diabetes Association. For information about Small Steps Press or the American Diabetes Association, in English or Spanish, call 1-800-342-2383. To order other Small Steps books, call 1-800-232-6733.

Every effort has been made by the author to include only recipes that have not been previously copyrighted. Should any such published recipe appear in this book, it is without her knowledge and is unintentional. The information and recipes in this book are not intended, nor should anything contained herein be construed, as an attempt to give, or be a substitute for medical advice or medical nutrition therapy. This book is not a medical manual and is not to be used as a substitute for treatment prescribed by your physician.

Consult a health care professional before trying any of the suggestions in this publication. Small Steps Press, ADA, and Brenda Ponichtera assume no responsibility for any injury that may result from the suggestions or information in this publication.

⊗ The paper in this publication meets the requirements of the ANSI Standard Z39.48-1992 (permanence of paper).

Small Steps Press titles may be purchased for business or promotional use or for special sales. To purchase bulk copies of this book at a discount, or for custom editions of this book with your logo, contact Small Steps Press at the address below, at booksales@diabetes.org, or by calling 703-299-2046.

For all other inquiries, please call 1-800-342-2383.

Small Steps Press
1701 North Beauregard Street
Alexandria, Virginia 22311

Library of Congress Cataloging-in-Publication Data
Ponichtera, Brenda J.
 Quick & healthy recipes and ideas : for people who say they don't have time to cook healthy meals / Brenda Ponichtera. -- 3rd ed.
    p. cm.
 Includes bibliographical references and index.
 ISBN 978-0-9816001-0-9 (alk. paper)
1. Low-cholesterol diet--Recipes. 2. Low-fat diet--Recipes. 3. Diabetes--Diet therapy--Recipes. 4. Low-carbohydrate diet--Recipes. 5. Quick and easy cookery. I. Title.

RM237.75.P65 2008
641.5'6383--dc22

2008022403

For more information visit http://www.QuickandHealthy.net.

To the three special men in my life,
my husband Ken, and my sons,
Kevin and Kyle

and

To the three special women in my life,
my mother, Mary Niemic, and my sisters,
Mary Lou Marques and Rosemary Gonneville.

Table of Contents

Acknowledgments

I could never do this alone. Thank you to the following for helping me to make this book a reality.

My husband, Ken—grocery shopper and recipe tester. Thanks for helping me survive another edition.

My sons, Kevin and Kyle, for your support and willingness to sample whatever I cook.

My administrative assistant, Nancy Taphouse, for your dedication to all my projects and your commitment to helping me do it right. I couldn't do it without you.

Lisa Becharas and Janice Staver, for sharing your creativeness over the years. You are both exceptional!

Bruno Amatter and Kate Bass, for so many years of support and dedication. I really appreciate both of you!

Madelyn L. Wheeler, MS, RD, CD, CDE, for going the extra mile to help me with recipe analysis and exchanges.

My support at the American Diabetes Association: Rob Anthony, Abe Ogden, and Heschel Falek for your patience and help along the way.

Recipe testers and recipe contributors, Claudia Schon, Nancy Taphouse, Carol Beer, Yvonne Lorenz, Jana and Rocky Webb, Ellie Timinsky, Sandra Fritz, Connie Christensen, Charlotte Johnson, Joyce Lehman, Debbie Kelly, Mike Newman, Jane Lyon, and Anita Clason.

The many professionals who have helped me along the way: Elizabeth Somer, MA, RD, Tracy Dugick, MS, RD, CDE, Karmeen Kulkarni, MS, RD, CDE, Kathy Isoldi, MS, RD, CDE, Hope S. Warshaw, MMSc, RD, CDE, Nancy Clark, MS, RD, Anne Daly, MS, RD, CDE, Kathy McManus, MS, RD, Kelly Chambers, MS, RD, CDE, Karen Deuster, MS, RD, Connie Evers, MS, RD, Bridget Swinney, MS, RD.

And lastly, to all of the people who use my cookbooks and have offered kind words of praise and stories of success—you have been my inspiration!

Preface

As in my previous books, my focus is health-conscious people who don't want to spend a lot of time in the kitchen. This includes families who want to eat more healthfully, people with diabetes or heart disease, and those wanting to lose weight.

With over 200 recipes to choose from, there is something for everyone. My emphasis is on low-fat, low-cholesterol, and high fiber, while limiting simple carbohydrates. Artificial sweeteners are included as an alternate to sugars when workable in the recipes.

In developing the recipes and all of the practical information in this book, I have kept in mind the following three goals that can lead to healthier living:

- Achieving and maintaining a desirable weight
- Eating more high-fiber carbohydrates and fewer simple carbohydrates
- Eating a low-fat diet (while using monounsaturated and polyunsaturated fats), limiting saturated fats, and avoiding *trans* fats

Each recipe includes diabetes and weight loss exchanges, nutrient analysis, and carb servings. The information not only helps those with dietary restrictions but also provides valuable information to the health-conscious consumer.

This book is more than a cookbook. I have also included practical nutrition guidelines, weight-loss tips, time-saving ideas, information on food products, and lots of menus. You'll find 20 weeks of dinner menus, each with a grocery list. Everything is designed to help you eat more healthfully and also save time.

Enjoy in good health!

Brenda J. Ponichtera,
Registered Dietitian

Recipe Notes

Sodium

Salt is listed as an optional ingredient in the recipes and is therefore not included in the nutrient analysis of the recipe. When using frozen or canned products, those with no salt added or reduced salt were used. If you are not accustomed to using sodium-reduced products, it may be more acceptable for your family if you make a gradual transition.

Fiber

Fiber is listed in the nutrient analysis of each recipe. Recipes that provide significant fiber also include one of the following notations:

- For 3–4 grams of fiber–One serving is a good source of fiber.

- For 5 or more grams of fiber–One serving is an excellent source of fiber.

Fiber Adjustment for Exchanges and Carb Servings

Carb servings and exchanges listed for the recipes have been adjusted for fiber. If the fiber is more than 5 grams, half of the grams of fiber are subtracted from the total grams of carbohydrate when figuring exchanges and carb servings. In some recipes, this resulted in no change.

Using Fresh Produce and Saving Time

Fresh produce is used in all recipes unless otherwise listed on the recipe as frozen or canned. If lack of time is keeping you from buying fresh vegetables, take advantage of produce that is cleaned, sliced, and/or peeled. Preparation time will be reduced considerably. See Time-Saving Ideas on page 19 for more helpful ways to save time.

Nutrient Analysis

If a choice of ingredients is given, the first one is used in the nutrient analysis. Optional ingredients are not included in the nutrient analysis. Figures have been rounded. If the value is less than .5, it is rounded down to zero. If the figure is .5 or more, it is rounded up to one. The following abbreviations are used in the nutrient analysis: g = grams, mg = milligrams. For a list of other measurements, conversions, and abbreviations used in this book, please refer to page 95.

Using Artificial Sweeteners

All brands of artificial sweeteners are not alike and you may prefer the taste of one over another. Some people note an undesirable aftertaste with some artificial sweeteners, but this seems to be an individual preference.

To offer another option for reducing calories and carbohydrates, we used artificial sweeteners as an alternative to sugars in a number of recipes. Listed below is what you can expect when using an artificial sweetener.

Non-Baked Recipes

Artificial sweeteners usually work well with foods that do not require baking. Cooking with artificial sweeteners is usually very acceptable if the recipe is not one that is expected to brown or rise.

Baked Recipes

Real sugar offers certain qualities to baked goods that artificial sweeteners do not. Real sugar helps baked goods to brown, contributes to the volume, adds moistness and tenderness, and helps the baked foods stay fresh longer.

You may note the following when artificial sweetener is used in place of all, or part, of the sugar:

- Cakes or muffins don't rise very well.
- The baked item does not brown.
- Baking time is often decreased.
- The flavor may need to be improved by adding vanilla extract.
- Baked goods will spoil more quickly if not stored in the refrigerator.

Some of the baked recipes in this book use artificial sweetener for part of the sugar. These recipes were considered acceptable by our recipe testing staff. However, the quality is not consistent with the same recipe made with all sugar and you may note some of the changes listed above. We did not use artificial sweeteners in recipes when the result was not acceptable.

NOTE: When using an artificial sweetener, refer to the label for the amount to substitute for sugar.

Food Exchanges for Diabetes and Weight Loss

Exchange lists are used in many weight-loss programs and diabetic diets. In forming the exchange lists, foods with similar calories, carbohydrate, protein, and fat are grouped together.

By following a meal pattern based on the exchange lists, one can "exchange" a food in one group for another food in the same group. This method helps to increase variety while at the same time keeping calories and nutrient values fairly consistent.

The basic exchange lists are:

Carbohydrates

Starch–includes breads, cereals, grains, starchy vegetables, and crackers

Fruit

Milk–includes milk and yogurt

Sweets, desserts, and other carbohydrates

Nonstarchy vegetables

Meat and Meat Substitutes (also includes cheese)

Lean

Medium-fat

High-fat

Plant-based proteins

Fats

The Meat and Meat Substitutes list and the Milk list are further divided into groups based on the amount of fat a food contains. The leanest meats and the fat-free/low-fat dairy products are the best choices.

Please be aware that the calories, carbohydrate, protein, and fat used for each exchange list are averages and are not always the exact values for a specific food within the exchange list.

Foods with less than 20 calories and 5 grams or less of carbohydrate per serving are listed as "free" for one serving. If you eat more than one serving, the food is not considered "free" and should be counted as an exchange.

Each recipe in this book has the exchanges listed. The figures used to calculate the exchanges are from *Choose Your Foods: Exchange Lists for Diabetes* by the American Diabetes Association and American Dietetic Association.

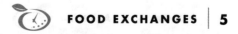

Carb Servings

All recipes in this book include Carb Servings, also known as Carb Choices. The general rule is 15 grams of carbohydrate equals 1 Carb Serving.

Talk to your registered dietitian or diabetes educator about adjusting the carbohydrate if a serving/portion of food has more than 5 grams of fiber.

NOTE: Carb servings and exchanges listed for the recipes have been adjusted for fiber. In some recipes, this resulted in no change. If the fiber is more than 5 grams, half of the grams of fiber are subtracted from the total grams of carbohydrate when figuring exchanges and carb servings.

The following chart was used to convert carbohydrate to Carb Servings.

Carbohydrate Grams	Carb Servings
0–5	0
6–10	1/2
11–20	1
21–25	1 1/2
26–35	2
36–40	2 1/2
41–50	3
51–55	3 1/2
56–65	4

Dietary Fiber

High-fiber foods should be part of your daily diet. Research has found that dietary fiber helps to lower cholesterol, improves blood sugar control, and protects against certain colon problems.

Two Types of Dietary Fiber

Insoluble fiber

This type of fiber is found in wheat bran, whole grains, and vegetables. It does not dissolve in water, but instead absorbs water. It provides bulk to stools and helps with bowel elimination. Studies indicate that this fiber may help to prevent problems associated with the colon, such as:

- Constipation
- Diverticulosis
- Hemorrhoids
- Colon and rectal cancer

Soluble fiber

This type of fiber is found in oats, legumes such as beans and peas, and some grains. It is also added to processed foods such as pectin and guar gums. It becomes a gel when mixed with water. Studies indicate that this fiber helps with:

- Lowering cholesterol by interfering with its production
- Improving blood sugar control by slowing the absorption of glucose

How much fiber do you need?

Your goal should be to consume at least 25 grams of dietary fiber every day. This is a real challenge for most people! The best sources of fiber are whole grains, fruits, vegetables, beans, and nuts.

Fiber is significantly reduced when fruits and vegetables are peeled and when grains are refined through processing.

- Foods with 2.5–4.9 grams of fiber are considered a good source.
- Foods with 5 or more grams of fiber are considered an excellent source.

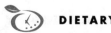

Sources of Dietary Fiber

Following is a listing of fiber sources and the approximate total grams of dietary fiber for the serving size listed. Use this as a guide but be sure to read labels on packaged foods, as the amount of fiber will vary with different brands.

Cereals	Fiber grams
All-Bran Buds, 1/3 cup	13
Bran Flakes, 3/4 cup	5
Cheerios, 1 cup	3
Fiber One, 1/2 cup	14
Frosted Mini-Wheats, 1 cup	6
Fruit & Fiber, 1 cup	5
Oatbran, 1 1/4 cups cooked	6
Oatmeal, 1 cup cooked	4
Oatmeal, instant, 1 packet	3
Raisin Bran, 1 cup	7
Shredded Wheat, 2 biscuits	5
Total, whole grain, 3/4 cup	3
Wheaties, 1 cup	3

Grains, Rice and Pasta	Fiber grams
Whole-wheat English muffin	4
Whole-grain bread, 1 ounce	3
Brown rice, 1/2 cup cooked	2
Barley, 1/2 cup cooked	3
Bulgur, 1/2 cup cooked	4
Spaghetti noodles, 1 cup cooked	2
Popcorn, 3 cups	3

Vegetables	Fiber grams
Asparagus, 1 cup cooked	3
Beets, 1/2 cup cooked	2
Broccoli, 1/2 cup cooked	3
Brussels sprouts, 1/2 cup cooked	2
Cauliflower, 1/2 cup cooked	2
Cabbage, 1/2 cup cooked	2
Carrots, 1/2 cup cooked	3
Corn, 1/2 cup cooked	2
Cucumber with peel, 1 medium	2
Eggplant, 1 cup cooked	3
Green beans, 1/2 cup cooked	2
Bell pepper, 1 medium raw	2
Potato, with skin, 1 medium	4
Snow peas, 1 cup raw	2
Spinach, 1/2 cup cooked	2
Summer squash, 1 cup cooked	3
Sweet potato, 1/2 cup cooked	3
Winter squash, 1/2 cup cooked	3

Dried Beans & Legumes	Fiber grams
Black beans, 1/2 cup cooked	8
Garbanzo, 1/2 cup cooked	6
Kidney beans, 1/2 cup cooked	6
Lentils, 1/2 cup cooked	8
Lima beans, 1/2 cup cooked	6
Pinto beans, 1/2 cup cooked	7
Peas, 1/2 cup cooked	4
Refried beans, fat-free, 1/2 cup	6
Split peas, 1/2 cup cooked	8

Fruits	Fiber grams
Apple with skin, 1 medium	4
Apricots, 5	4
Avocado, 1 medium*	9
Banana, 1 medium	3
Blueberries, 1 cup	4
Cherries, 1 cup	3
Grapefruit, 1 medium	3
Grapes, seedless, 1 cup	2
Kiwi, 1 medium	3
Nectarine, 1 medium	2
Orange, 1 medium	3
Peach, 1 medium	2
Pear, 1 medium	4
Pineapple, 1 cup	2
Plums, 2	2
Prunes, dried, 5	3
Raisins, 1/4 cup	2
Raspberries, 1 cup	8
Strawberries, 1 cup	3

Nuts/Seeds, dry roasted*	Fiber grams
Almonds, 24 nuts (1 ounce)	3
Cashews, 18 nuts (1 ounce)	1
Filberts (hazelnuts), 20 nuts	3
Flaxseeds, 1 tablespoon	3
Peanuts, 28 nuts (1 ounce)	2
Pistachios, 47 nuts (1 ounce)	3
Soy nuts, 1/4 cup (1 1/2 ounces)	3
Sunflower seeds, kernels, (1 ounce)	3
Walnuts, 14 halves (1 ounce)	2
Peanut butter, 2 tablespoons	2

Although these foods are higher in fat, most of the fat is healthy monounsaturated and polyunsaturated.

Tips for Reducing Fat and Cholesterol in Your Diet

Limiting fat and cholesterol in your diet is important, whether your goal is to lose weight, lower your cholesterol, or just be more healthy. Here are some ideas to help.

Substitute low-fat snacks for high-fat snacks and limit the amount you eat.

Look for no more than 3 grams of fat for every 100 calories. Avoid any with *trans* fats. The following foods are good options:

- 1 ounce of nuts*
- fresh fruit
- fat-free hot cocoa
- low-fat frozen yogurt
- low-fat ice milk
- low-fat crackers and cookies
- rice cakes
- frozen juice bars
- unsalted-top saltines
- air-popped popcorn
- pretzels, both hard and soft
- tomato juice with a twist of lemon
- corn cakes (caramel flavor is a favorite)
- fruit slices served with fat-free yogurt for dipping

- graham crackers, vanilla wafers, gingersnaps, animal crackers, fig bars
- soda pop with a scoop of low-fat ice milk (use diet pop to reduce calories)
- light microwave popcorn, butter flavor or kettle corn
- raw vegetable sticks with low-fat ranch dressing for a dip

Nuts are a good choice because they contain heart-healthy monounsaturated and/or polyunsaturated fat. Limit to 1 ounce a day.

Change how you prepare foods.

- Remove the skin from chicken.
- Remove fat from homemade and canned soups.
- Bake, broil, simmer, microwave, or barbecue.
- Cook foods in a few tablespoons of broth, fruit juice, or water.
- When frying foods, use nonstick cooking spray or use a spray pump.

Substitute the following lower-fat or fat-free foods for higher-fat foods.

- Fat-free or 1% milk
- Evaporated skim milk
- Fat-free yogurt (plain or flavored)
- Ice milk
- Light, reduced-fat, or fat-free sour cream
- Light, reduced-fat, or fat-free cream cheese
- Low-fat, reduced-fat, or fat-free mayonnaise
- Low-fat, reduced-fat, or fat-free salad dressings
- Low-fat or reduced-fat cheeses
- Low-fat or reduced-fat margarine
- Water-packed tuna

Avoid or limit the following foods.

- High-fat meats such as bacon, bologna, and salami
- Foods fried in oil, lard, or other fats
- Fried snack foods, such as potato chips, corn chips, and cheese curls
- Pastries, cookies, and rich desserts
- Foods with *trans* fats (these are foods that list hydrogenated or partially hydrogenated in the list of ingredients)

Choose the following.

- Only lean meats and cut off all fat before cooking
- Lean beef with 7% fat or less
- Ground turkey with 7% fat or less
- Meat that has little or no marbling of fat
- An egg substitute to limit egg yolks, or use two egg whites in place of one egg
- A sprinkle of imitation butter flavor sprinkles instead of margarine on vegetables
- A fruit spread or fat-free cream cheese on toast instead of margarine
- Lettuce and tomato on sandwiches and leave off the mayonnaise
- A margarine that does not have *trans* fats

Most fruits and vegetables are fat-free and are good low-calorie, high-fiber choices. Your higher-fat foods are often processed foods such as fried foods, frozen breaded products, cookies, pastries, chips, and fast foods. Cutting back on fat and eating more fruits and vegetables is also a good way to lose weight.

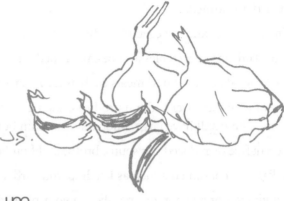

Reducing Sodium

Not everyone needs to be on a sodium-restricted diet. However, it is still prudent to limit sodium to no more than 2300 milligrams per day. If you are on a sodium-restricted diet, you may find it helpful to seek guidance from a registered dietitian.

The three best ways to cut back on sodium

1. **Don't use salt at the table.**

2. **Use less salt in cooking.**
   Keep in mind that a small amount used in cooking may give just enough flavor to help you from adding too much at the table.

3. **Avoid processed foods.**
   These are convenience foods, canned foods, fast foods, and most snack foods. Processed foods usually have salt added and have more sodium than fresh foods.

If you are trying to reduce the sodium in your diet, here are some additional guidelines

- Use fresh foods in place of processed foods when possible.

- Buy frozen vegetables when possible. Most have no salt added and they also taste better than canned.

- When buying canned vegetables, choose those with no added salt.

- Drain and rinse vegetables and beans canned with salt.

- Don't eat salted and cured meats such as ham, bacon, and luncheon meats.

- Try some of the lower sodium products, such as reduced-salt ham or reduced-salt bacon. These still have large amounts of sodium but less than the real thing.

- Use salt-free or reduced-salt soups, broth, and bouillon.

- Go light on condiments such as ketchup, mustard, and steak sauce.

- Add vinegar or a lemon or lime slice to your plate to flavor fish and vegetables such as spinach.

- Use seasoning powders and do not use seasoning salts. Garlic powder is a better choice than garlic salt.

- Learn to use herbs and spices in cooking to add flavor. Herbs and spices are not a significant source of sodium.

- Try unsalted snack foods, such as:
  - unsalted, baked tortilla chips
  - unsalted popcorn
  - whole-grain crackers with unsalted tops

- Make fast foods lower in sodium by ordering hamburgers without pickles and cheese. Order French fries without salt.

NOTE: Salt is listed as an optional ingredient in the recipes in this book and is therefore not included in the nutrient analysis of the recipes. When possible, frozen or canned products without the addition of salt, or reduced salt, were used. If you are not accustomed to using sodium-reduced products, it may be more acceptable for your family if you make a gradual transition.

Ten Steps to Weight Loss

If your goal is to lose weight, try some of these helpful ideas:

1. ## Plan
   - Plan meals before shopping.
   - Make a grocery list.
   - Grocery shop when you are NOT hungry.
   - Do not buy high-calorie foods that you will be too tempted to eat.

2. ## Make better food choices
   - Choose low-fat foods and high-fiber foods.
   - Use less fat in cooking.
   - Try recipes that are low fat and low calorie.
   - Use less foods that are high in saturated fats.
   - Avoid foods with *trans* fats.
   - Replace saturated fats and *trans* fats with monounsaturated and polyunsaturated fats. (See page 10 for information on fats.)

3. ## Eat less
   - Eat a smaller amount. This is just as important as what you eat.
   - Portion control is the key to long-term weight loss.
   - Cook only the amount you need if you are tempted by leftovers.
   - Use a smaller plate so it will not look empty.

4. ## Control snacking
   - Have lower-calorie snacks on hand, such as fresh fruit, vegetables, and diet soda pop.
   - Try 1 ounce of nuts.
   - Limit how often you snack and eat smaller amounts.
   - Ask yourself if you are hungry. Only eat if hungry.

5. ## Keep food out of sight
   - Never leave food on the counter.
   - Store it out of sight behind a cupboard door.
   - Put tempting food in hard-to-reach places.

6. Don't eat just for something to do
   - Find a hobby you enjoy.
   - Go for a walk.
   - Call or visit a friend.
   - Do volunteer work.
   - Get a job.

7. Change your eating habits
   - Make a list of your bad eating habits.
   - Write down what you can do to change each bad habit.
   - Practice good eating habits.

8. Set a goal you can reach
   - Be realistic.
   - A 1- to 2-pound loss per week is good.
   - Choose a weight goal that is good for you.
   - Consult a registered dietitian for goal setting and for advice on meal planning and a weight loss plan.

9. Exercise
   - Exercise every day or at least four to five times a week.
   - Start slowly and build up gradually.
   - Find a friend to walk with.
   - Choose a time of the day that is good for you.

   (See pages 17–18 for more information on exercise.)

10. Enjoy eating
   - Eat slowly and enjoy each bite.
   - Do not drink when there is food in your mouth.
   - Put your fork down while chewing and only pick it up when your mouth is empty.
   - Do nothing else while eating so you can enjoy each bite.
   - A smaller amount of food eaten slowly can be more enjoyable than a larger amount eaten fast.

Exercise—Get Going!

Exercising for 60 minutes every day should be your goal. However, exercising just 20–30 minutes, four to five times a week, is also very good. Anything you do to get your body moving is better than doing nothing at all. Start slowly and build up gradually. Also consider the exercise you get while cleaning house, doing yard work, going up and down stairs, etc. It all adds up.

NOTE: It is very important to consult a physician before starting any exercise program.

Some of the popular aerobic exercises—exercise that uses oxygen—are walking, jogging, aerobic classes, jumping rope, and use of special equipment such as a stair stepper, elliptical trainer, cross-country machine, and treadmill.

The Benefits of Exercise

- Lowers risk of heart disease
- Increases good cholesterol
- Improves blood pressure
- Lowers risk of osteoporosis
- Improves blood sugar control

- Increases basal metabolic rate
- Helps with weight loss
- Lowers body fat
- Improves quality of life
- Improves mental health and reduces depression

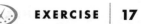

Some Ideas to Get You Started

Do what you enjoy
If you enjoy what you are doing, there is a better chance you will continue.

Get a routine going
Plan to exercise every day. If you miss one day you will still have exercised six days that week. Exercising on a regular basis becomes a routine—like brushing your teeth.

Find a time that works for you
Look at your daily schedule and see what time of the day is good for you.

Ask friends to join you
Exercising with friends will make the time go by faster and it's more fun.

Have a back-up plan
If you won't walk in the rain, plan to walk in a mall or go to a health club. If you go to exercise classes and know you will miss one, plan on doing another kind of exercise at a better time for you.

Wear the right shoes and clothing
If you walk for exercise, you'll need good walking shoes and a raincoat. Sweat suits or shorts are fine for health clubs. You don't have to buy expensive clothes.

Don't put off exercising until tomorrow
Remember, tomorrow never comes.

Add extra steps throughout your day
Park the car further away, use stairs instead of elevators, and walk during your break time. Every little bit counts.

You are important
Your health, both physical and mental, is important. It's okay to take time for yourself to exercise or just to relax. Don't feel guilty!

Think positive and you will succeed!

 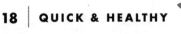

Time-Saving Ideas

Ideas to Help You Save Time in the Kitchen

Take advantage of produce that is cleaned, sliced, and/or peeled. Although these may cost more, it is worth it if lack of time is keeping you from eating fresh vegetables.

Buy whole vegetables—including lettuce—that have not been cleaned or sliced. Save time by cleaning and slicing the vegetables, all at one time, and then refrigerate in resealable plastic bags. This will be less expensive.

A salad spinner is a must to make cleaning lettuce a quick task. Do a whole head of lettuce and store in resealable plastic bags. I prefer this type of lettuce over the packages of pre-washed lettuce.

Use alfalfa sprouts in sandwiches and salads. These are ready to use right from the container. No chopping!

Buy packages of stir-fry vegetables and meat or poultry ready cut for stir-frying.

Stock your freezer with foods that thaw quickly for last-minute meals. An example is packages of individually frozen skinned and boned chicken breasts. However, check the label for sodium, as many have salt added.

To skin chicken parts, place a paper towel on the skin and pull.

Purchase packaged cornflake crumbs, instead of crushing cornflakes, for use in breading meats. These are usually found with the breadings in the grocery store.

Use quick-cooking brown rice. It cooks in only 10 minutes!

Chopping cilantro can be simplified. Save time and reduce spoilage by chopping a bunch at one time and freezing for future use. Fresh is best, but frozen also works well in recipes. Wash a bunch of cilantro with the stems tied together. Shake off water. Start chopping from the leafy end—on a cutting board—and stop chopping when you reach mostly stems. A French knife works well for this task. Freeze in resealable plastic bags. Small amounts can easily be removed as needed.

Fresh herbs always taste the best, but dried herbs also work well. When buying fresh, chop all at one time and freeze in resealable plastic bags for future use.

The taste of fresh minced ginger is hard to replace. If not using within a week, freeze for future use. Save time by mincing all at one time and freezing in resealable plastic bags. Or freeze the ginger whole and grate the amount you need, while frozen.

Purchase chopped or minced garlic in a jar and substitute it for fresh. It's available in the produce section. This saves time chopping.

Use dried onion instead of chopping fresh. See the label for reconstituting.

Marinate foods in a resealable plastic bag. This eliminates extra clean-up. Always marinate meat, poultry, and seafood in the refrigerator.

Keep staple foods on hand so that you always have the ingredients for several meals.

Organize your grocery list in categories so you will be less likely to miss an item. Find a convenient place in your kitchen for the list and encourage family members to add to it. Ask them to add items when they are low and not empty.

Plan meals for the next week and add items needed to the grocery list before shopping.

Grocery shop from your list once a week and avoid stops at the grocery store after work.

Cook once and serve twice. Double a recipe and freeze for future meals or freeze in individual portions for lunch.

Products Worth Trying

Listed below are some products, with a brief description, that are worth trying. Although brand names may be mentioned, there are probably other brands with similar nutrient values.

Fresh Chopped or Minced Garlic: You'll find it in a jar and in the produce section of the grocery store. Use 1/2 teaspoon in place of one garlic clove.

Dried Chopped Onion: This is sold in the section with seasonings and herbs. Use 2 tablespoons to replace 1/2 cup chopped raw onion.

Rice Vinegar: Rice vinegar is very good on salads. Sweeten with sugar or artificial sweetener to taste. One tablespoon is 0 calories.

Balsamic Vinegar: This very flavorful vinegar can be used on salads without the addition of other ingredients. One tablespoon is 10 calories.

Lite Soy Sauce: Most have 50% less sodium than regular soy sauce. Or you can dilute regular soy sauce with an equal amount of water to reduce the sodium. One-half teaspoon of the regular, diluted with an equal amount of water, has 153 milligrams of sodium. An equal amount of the lite version (1 teaspoon) has 190 milligrams of sodium, and the diluted regular soy sauce actually tastes better than the lite.

Butter-Flavored Sprinkles: These are good sprinkled on vegetables. One-half teaspoon contains 4 calories and 90 milligrams of sodium.

Hickory Liquid Smoke: Just a drop adds a very good smoky flavor. Good in marinades. Found by the barbecue sauce in the grocery store.

Ground Fresh Chili Paste: Adds hot spiciness to Asian dishes. You use just a small amount and it keeps well in the refrigerator after opening. Available in the Asian foods section of the grocery store.

Lite Coconut Milk: A flavorful ingredient used in Thai foods. Be sure to buy the lite version and to limit your portion, as it is still high in fat. Available in the Asian foods section of the grocery store.

Nonstick Cooking Spray: Use for frying without adding extra calories. Or buy a spray pump and fill it will olive or canola oil. Just pump and spray.

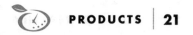

Canola Oil: This oil contains the least amount of saturated fat and the most amount of monounsaturated fat. A very good choice.

Olive Oil: This flavorful oil is high in monounsaturated fat and is a very good choice. The extra virgin has the strongest flavor and is the one I prefer.

Sesame Oil: This is another oil high in monounsaturated fat. It has a distinct flavor that is very good in salads, in sauces, and for stir-frying. Store in the refrigerator after opening to preserve freshness.

Light Mayonnaise: A good choice. One tablespoon contains about 50 calories.

Fat-Free Mayonnaise: The flavor is too bland but it can be spiced up with a small amount of mustard or vinegar.

Fat-Free Yogurts: Choose from plain, sweetened with sugar, or sweetened with artificial sweetener. Calories vary from 80 to 150 for 6–8 ounces.

Fat-Free Sour Cream: There are several good brands on the market. These have a good flavor, as good as the regular, and have only 10 calories for one tablespoon!

Evaporated Fat-Free Milk: Use in baking, especially when making pumpkin pie (with or without a crust). It tastes very good and you won't miss the fat or the extra calories. This product has 25 calories per 2 tablespoons, versus 40 calories in the regular.

Fat-Free Half and Half: This a good substitute for the high-fat version. Two tablespoons have 20 calories, 0 grams fat, and 3 grams of carbohydrate.

Salad Dressings: Many are available that are lower in fat or fat-free. Have a variety on hand.

Salad Spritzers: Only 10 calories for 10 sprays. Available in a variety of flavors. A really good choice to limit the amount of salad dressing that you use.

Quick-Cooking Brown Rice: Cooks in only 10 minutes!

Spaghetti Sauce: Look for less than 4 grams of fat for 4 ounces.

Egg Substitute: This product can be found in the refrigerated section of the grocery store. These are a good choice for limiting whole eggs. Most products are fat-free and have only 30 calories for 1/4 cup.

 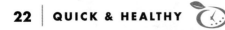

Cheese: Many low-fat and reduced-fat varieties are now on the market. I prefer to buy the ones that are called reduced-fat with 3–5 grams of fat per ounce. These seem to taste better than those lower in fat and they also melt more like regular cheese.

- **Laughing Cow Light Cheese:** This spreadable cheese is available in a variety of light flavors. Each 3/4-ounce wedge contains 2 grams of fat, 35 calories, and 260 milligrams of sodium.

- **Fat-Free Feta Cheese:** Surprisingly, this has a great flavor and only 30 calories for 1 ounce! This should be limited by those on a sodium-restricted diet, as it has 450 milligrams of sodium for 1 ounce.

- **Parmesan Cheese:** The flavor of fresh is far better than the grated you purchase in a can. Available in the deli section of your local grocery store, either grated or whole. Inexpensive hand graters are also available. Limit your portion, as the fat can add up.

- **Light Cream Cheese and Fat-Free Cream Cheese:** These are a good replacement for regular cream cheese. The light contains about half the fat and about 30 calories for 1 tablespoon. The fat-free has only 15 calories for 1 tablespoon. Although the light has a better flavor and texture, limit your portions, as the fat can easily add up. When the cream cheese is a predominate flavor in the recipe, you may prefer to use the light or half of each type.

Fat-Free Refried Beans: An excellent source of fiber with no fat.

Low-Fat Canned Chili: Several brands are available that meet the goal of no more than 30% of the calories from fat. Check the label and look for those with no more than 8 grams of fat per 240 calories (usually 1/2 can). An excellent source of fiber.

Packages of Individually Frozen, Skinned, and Boned Chicken Breasts or Chicken Tenderloins: The tenderloins are the most tender part of the breast and what I often use. These convenient packages allow you to easily remove the number of pieces you want without having to thaw the whole package. Check the sodium on the label as some have salt added.

Ground Turkey: Look for packages of lean ground turkey that have only 7% fat. Be aware that much of the ground turkey sold contains 15% fat.

Ground Beef: Choose the very lean ground beef with only 7% fat.

Smoked Turkey Sausage: This looks like and tastes like Polish kielbasa, but it is much lower in fat. It is still high in sodium, so limit the amount.

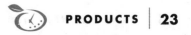 **PRODUCTS** | **23**

Frozen TV Dinners: When choosing a TV dinner, look for those with less than 800 milligrams of sodium and fat providing no more than 30% of the calories. If the dinner is about 300 calories, the fat should be 10 grams or less.

Canned Soups: There are several brands that have low-fat or fat-free soups and some that are also lower in sodium. Choose soups that are 98% fat-free.

Swanson Broths: These have a good flavor and can replace homemade broth. Both the chicken and beef are available fat-free and reduced sodium. Available in 14.5-ounce cans and 32-ounce boxes.

Au Jus Gravy Mix: This is a good product to use when making French dip sandwiches. I prefer French's brand, which can be found with the packaged gravies and sauces. To reduce the sodium, dilute with more water.

Country Gravy Mix: This is a bit high in sodium but still a good choice if you limit the amount. We used it in our Biscuits and Gravy recipe, page 305. You'll find this product with all of the packaged gravy mixes. One-fourth of a cup is 40 calories, 2 grams of fat, 0 grams saturated fat, 0 grams *trans* fat, 280 milligrams sodium, and 5 grams of carbohydrate. Several good brands are available and we found the low-fat had the same fat content as the regular. Check the label and compare with what is listed here.

Packaged Coleslaw Vegetables: Just add dressing. No chopping!

Alfalfa Sprouts: Great in sandwiches! These are ready to use right from the container.

Yukon Gold Potatoes: These are new potatoes with an excellent flavor. Simply slice, season to taste, and cook in a covered casserole in the oven or in the microwave.

Fat-Free Whipped Topping: Available in the freezer section. Only 15 calories for two tablespoons.

Sugar-Free, Fat-Free Pudding Mixes: These are fat-free if made with fat-free milk and are available both in the cooked version and instant. The instant can be prepared in just minutes. Most are about 70 calories for one serving when made with nonfat milk. These are used in several of the dessert recipes in this book and they have the texture of a rich mousse.

Sugar-Free Gelatin: A good low-calorie choice for a dessert. Only ten calories in 1/2 cup! There are a variety of flavors and they take little time to prepare.

 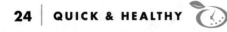

Frozen Dessert Bars: Look for those with 80 calories or less. Some are sweetened with sugar, while some are sweetened with artificial sweetener. Avoid those that contain palm oil or coconut oil. Some popsicles have only 14 calories!

Fat-Free Hot Cocoa Mix: Only 25 calories and 5 grams of carbohydrate per cup.

Flavored Seltzer Water: There are several brands available with a variety of flavors sweetened with artificial sweetener. These remind me of a "sophisticated" diet soda. Strawberry is my favorite flavor. Be sure to check the labels for the sugar-free version. Most have 0 calories.

Crystal Light Beverage: This product is a powder that you mix with water to make a refreshing drink. It's great on a hot summer day. There are several very good flavors including lemonade, which is my favorite. It is sweetened with artificial sweetener and has only 5 calories for an 8-ounce drink.

Cornflake Crumbs: You don't have to crush cornflakes to make crumbs. You can buy packaged crumbs in the grocery; they're usually found by the breadings and not with the cereals.

Biscuits: We found the store brand of ready-to-bake biscuits were an okay choice. Still not as good a choice as a whole-grain roll, but if you need biscuits for a recipe, these are worth trying. When searching in your grocery store, look for those that are only 100 calories, 1.5 grams of fat, and 1 gram of fiber for two biscuits. Be sure to check labels, as many are higher in fat and have no fiber.

Whole-Grain Breads and Rolls: Choose those with 3 grams of fiber and no more than 2 grams of fat per serving. A good source of fiber.

Baked Chips: If you are missing potato chips, check the label on the baked version, as you can find these with no *trans* fats and almost no fat. The sodium is still significant. About 110 calories in 1 ounce, which is about 11 chips. Still limit your serving.

Sugar-Free Maple Syrup: This is also known as breakfast syrup and is available in several brands. Very acceptable flavor.

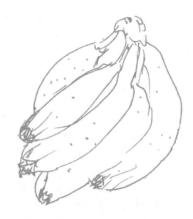

Quick Ideas for Meals— No Recipes Needed!

Quick Breakfast Ideas

A good breakfast gives you a jump-start for the day. It provides energy as well as valuable nutrients. Include some of the following for a healthy breakfast:

- **Protein-rich foods**–Choose those low in fat such as lean meats, low-fat cheeses, and egg substitute (or eggs within recommended amount).
- **Fresh fruit or fruit juice**–Fresh fruit is a better choice, as it provides more fiber than juice.
- **Whole-grain breads and cereals**–These add fiber to your diet.
- **Fat-free dairy products**–Choose fat-free milk or yogurt.

Breakfast ideas that do not require a recipe

Hot Cereal
Cook oatmeal or oat bran cereal. Top with fat-free or low-fat yogurt and fruit.

Cold Cereal
Serve whole-grain cereal with fat-free milk and fresh fruit. Look for cereal with less than 3 grams of fat per serving and at least 3 grams of fiber per serving.

 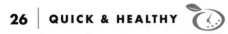

Peanut Butter
Spread on whole-grain toast.

Bagel
Top a whole-grain bagel with fat-free or low-fat cream cheese or a low-fat, spreadable cheese.

Yogurt and Fruit
Add fruit to fat-free or low-fat yogurt. Fresh berries work well and add fiber. Serve with whole-grain toast.

Breakfast Yogurt
Mix fat-free or low-fat yogurt with fresh fruit. Add a high-fiber cereal.

Breakfast Pizza
Toast a whole-grain English muffin half. Top with pizza sauce (or tomato sauce or chili sauce) and reduced-fat mozzarella cheese. Heat under broiler until cheese is melted.

Omelets
Make an omelet and top with salsa. Egg substitute works well in omelets. Add cooked mushrooms or other vegetables. This is a good way to use leftover vegetables.

Low-Fat Cooking
Use nonstick cooking spray for cooking tortillas, pancakes, French toast, and eggs or egg substitute.

Reduce Fat
Try whole-wheat toast with sugar-free jam and leave off the margarine.

Low-Sugar
Use sugar-free jam on pancakes or French toast. Unsweetened applesauce is also good on pancakes.

Cheese and Fruit
Serve low-fat cottage cheese or low-fat ricotta cheese with fruit. Add whole-grain toast.

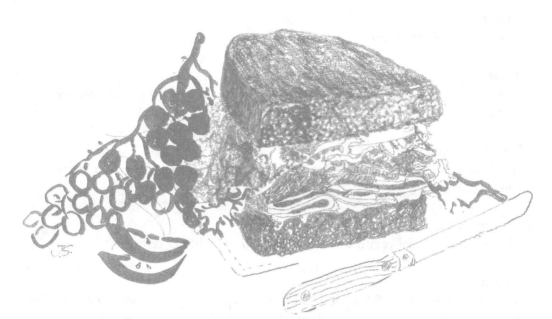

Quick Cold Sandwich Ideas

Ideas for variety, saving time, and cutting calories and fat

Add Moisture

Cut back on calories by using a light mayonnaise spread thinly. Or leave off the mayonnaise or margarine and use one of the following for moisture:

- Whole, canned green chiles–cut lengthwise
- Lettuce and tomato
- Sweet or mild onion
- Avocado slices–avocado is an excellent source of fiber and a rich source of heart-healthy monounsaturated fats

Coleslaw

Try well-drained coleslaw in a sandwich for crunch and moisture.

Alfalfa Sprouts

Use in place of lettuce; they don't get soggy.

 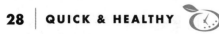

Pita Bread Pockets

Cut a whole-grain pita bread in half. Fill with raw vegetables and tuna salad or lean sliced turkey.

Rice Cakes

Top with low-fat ricotta cheese and salsa, or low-fat ricotta cheese and a sprinkle of cinnamon and sugar (or artificial sweetener).

Submarine Sandwich

Layer on a whole-grain roll lean meat, poultry, or seafood; low-fat or reduced-fat cheese; sliced onion; and chopped lettuce. Use a fat-free or low-fat Italian dressing on the lettuce.

Tuna Salad with a Different Flavor

Mix water-packed tuna (drained) and light mayonnaise, add 1 tablespoon of pickle relish or diced green chiles, and add some chopped celery for crunch.

Cream Cheese

Spread a thin layer of cream cheese (light or fat-free) on whole-wheat bread or a bagel. Add slices of lean meat, such as smoked turkey or lean roast beef, and top with sprouts or lettuce.

Turkey Special

On your favorite whole-grain bread, layer sliced turkey, cream cheese (light or fat-free), cranberry sauce, and sprouts.

Deli Wrap

Layer lean meat and low-fat or reduced-fat cheese on a flavored tortilla wrap. Add some of the following:

- Tomatoes
- Relishes
- Cranberry sauce
- Plain or flavored cream cheese (low-fat or fat-free)
- Chopped lettuce and/or sprouts

Roll up for a tasty sandwich.

Quick Hot Sandwich Ideas

Reuben Sandwich
On whole-wheat toast, layer smoked turkey, sauerkraut (rinsed twice and well drained), and reduced-fat mozzarella cheese. Heat under broiler until cheese is melted. Top with a slice of toast or serve open-faced.

French Dip
Use thinly sliced lean roast beef or turkey on a whole-grain roll. For dipping, make au jus gravy mix using package directions (you can cut back on the sodium by adding more water when making the au jus).

Individual Pizza
Toast a whole-grain English muffin half and top with pizza sauce (or tomato sauce or chili sauce) and reduced-fat mozzarella cheese. Heat under broiler until cheese is melted.

Chicken Barbecue Sandwich
Microwave (or cook in a skillet) a chicken breast, without bone or skin—be sure to cook until chicken is no longer pink. Serve on a whole-grain bun and top with lettuce, a tomato slice, and barbecue sauce.

Hot Pita Sandwich
Spray a skillet with nonstick cooking spray. Over medium heat, cook chopped lean meat (or poultry or seafood) and vegetables until meat is done and vegetables are tender. Cut whole-grain pita bread in half and fill with cooked meat and vegetables.

Tacos
Fill a heated whole-wheat flour or corn tortilla with fat-free refried beans and/or chopped cooked lean meat or poultry. Finish with chopped lettuce, tomato, onion, and salsa.

Quesadilla
Top a whole-wheat flour tortilla with a small amount of cooked lean meat and low-fat or reduced-fat grated cheese (you can also add drained chiles and chopped green onion). Cover with another tortilla. Spray a skillet with nonstick cooking spray and, over medium heat, brown on both sides until cheese is melted.

Quick Ideas for Lunch and Dinner

Shish Kebab
Make by skewering any or all of the following:

- Green peppers pieces
- Onion quarters
- Canned new potatoes
- Cubes of lean meat, poultry, or shrimp

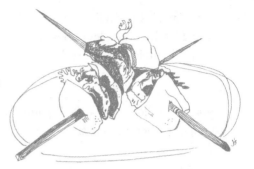

Broil or barbecue until done.

Baked Stuffed Potato
Split and fill with one of the following:

- Low-fat cottage cheese and chopped green onion
- Black beans and salsa
- Low-fat canned chili* and chopped onion

Cold Plate
Make a cold plate using either low-fat cottage cheese with sliced fruit (fresh or canned without sugar); OR sliced lean meats, low-fat or reduced-fat cheese, and raw vegetables. Add a whole-grain roll or unsalted top crackers.

Tossed Salads
Top with kidney or garbanzo beans for protein.

Macaroni and Cheese
Make macaroni and cheese from the box using fat-free milk and leave out (or cut back on) the margarine.

Burrito
On a heated whole-wheat tortilla, layer fat-free refried beans or black beans, low-fat or reduced-fat grated cheese, chopped lettuce, and tomatoes. Roll up and serve with salsa and fat-free sour cream.

Low-fat canned chili has no more than 8 grams of fat per 240 calories

Chili

Serve a low-fat canned chili*. Top with grated low-fat or reduced-fat cheese and sliced green onion. Serve with raw carrot and celery sticks.

Stir-Fry

Make a simple meal! Brown lean meat, seafood, or poultry, and then add a couple of sliced/chopped fresh vegetables. Cook until done. Serve with cooked rice or noodles, or serve in a heated whole-wheat tortilla.

Spaghetti

Serve spaghetti noodles with bottled spaghetti sauce. Choose a spaghetti sauce with less than 4 grams of fat per 4 ounces.

*Low-fat canned chili has no more than 8 grams of fat per 240 calories

 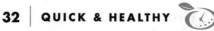

Quick Ideas for Desserts

Angel Food Cake
Top with fresh fruit and fat-free whipped topping.

Frozen Dessert
Start with angel food cake and fat-free or low-fat frozen yogurt. Slice the cake horizontally into three layers. Spread softened frozen yogurt between each layer. Freeze until 10 minutes before serving.

Filled Cantaloupe
Cut cantaloupe in half and scoop out seeds. Fill the center with fruit-flavored gelatin* (make following package directions) and refrigerate until set. Cut in half before serving.

Topping
Top fruit-flavored gelatin* (make following package directions) with fat-free or low-fat vanilla or lemon yogurt*.

Fruit Slush
Start with about 1 cup of frozen sliced fruit. Add to blender with about 1/2 cup fat-free milk or yogurt*. Blend until smooth and then sweeten to taste.

Fruit Platter
Place sliced fresh fruit on a plate. Serve with a bowl of fat-free or low-fat yogurt* to serve as a dip or topping.

Frozen Fruit Bars*
Many choices are in the grocery store. Look for those with less than 80 calories and no fat.

Frosting
Frost a cake with fat-free whipped topping.

Layered Dessert
Layer fruit-flavored gelatin* with pudding* in parfait or clear glasses. Use package directions to make both the gelatin and pudding using fat-free milk in the pudding.

Use sugar-free options to reduce carbohydrate and limit calories.

Getting Organized

Saving time starts with planning. If you plan your meals for the week, use a grocery list divided into categories to help you stay organized. It is especially helpful when you are shopping so you won't miss items that you intend to buy. Follow our sample grocery list on page 35 and make copies to use. Save more time by using the weekly menus in this book—20 weeks in all. Each comes with a complete grocery list.

Grocery List Tips

- Find a convenient place in your kitchen for your grocery list. Encourage family members to add to it.

- Add items to your list when they are low and not empty; that way you never run out.

- Plan meals for the next week and add the items needed to the grocery list before shopping.

- Grocery shop from your grocery list once a week and avoid stops to the grocery store after work or at dinnertime when it seems to be the busiest.

- Never shop when hungry. This is when you'll be most tempted to make poor choices.

Stocking Your Pantry

Having a well-stocked pantry will save you time. These are usually nonperishable items you want on hand so you can put together a meal in a moment's notice. Also, having these items readily available will prevent needless stops to the grocery store.

The staple grocery list on page 36 has items that have a longer shelf life. Many of these may already be in your home. You may prefer to purchase in larger quantities so you won't have to shop for these items weekly.

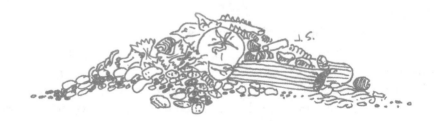

Weekly Grocery List

Canned Fruits & Juices

_____

_____

_____

Canned Vegetables, Sauces, & Soups

_____

_____

_____

Pasta, Rice, & Beans

_____

_____

_____

Breads & Cereals

_____

_____

_____

Fresh Produce

_____

_____

_____

Dairy & Cheese

_____

_____

_____

Miscellaneous

_____

_____

_____

Meat, Poultry, & Seafood

_____

_____

_____

Frozen Foods

_____

_____

_____

Paper & Cleaning Products

_____

_____

_____

Grocery List: Staples

Spices & Seasonings

anise seed
bay leaves
cayenne pepper
celery seed
chili powder
crushed red pepper
curry powder
dried basil
dried cilantro
dried dill weed
dried marjoram
dried minced onion
dried oregano
dried parsley
dried rosemary
dried sage
dried tarragon
dried thyme
fat-free butter-flavored sprinkles
fennel seed
fresh or jar of chopped/minced garlic
garlic powder
ground allspice
ground black pepper
ground cinnamon
ground cloves
ground cumin
ground ginger
ground mustard
ground nutmeg
Italian seasoning
onion powder
paprika
poppy seeds
salt (optional)
toasted sesame seeds

Baking Products

baking powder
baking soda
cornstarch
instant chicken bouillon
artificial sweetener
brown sugar
granulated sugar
honey
molasses
nonstick cooking spray
canola oil
olive oil
sesame oil
pudding, sugar free, instant (chocolate, vanilla, white chocolate, cheesecake)
gelatin, sugar free, fruit flavored (lime, raspberry, lemon)
unbleached all-purpose flour
whole-wheat flour
almond extract
peppermint extract
vanilla extract

Dressings, Sauces, Jams, & Vinegar

apple cider vinegar
red wine vinegar
rice vinegar
barbecue sauce
catsup
hickory liquid smoke (found by the barbecue sauce)
Dijon mustard
prepared mustard
light mayonnaise
Miracle Whip Light
reduced-fat or fat-free salad dressing
Tabasco sauce
Worcestershire sauce
dry sherry

Canned Vegetables/Sauces/Soups

To lower sodium, choose no added salt or reduced sodium.

beef broth, fat free
chicken broth, fat free
cream of celery soup, low fat, condensed
cream of chicken soup, low fat, condensed
cream of mushroom soup, low fat, condensed
tomato soup, condensed
artichoke hearts, quartered
creamed corn
mushroom pieces and stems
pimiento, chopped
pinto beans
sauerkraut
tomato juice
tomatoes, diced, stewed
tomato sauce
pizza sauce
spaghetti sauce (less than 4 g fat per 4 oz)
black-eyed peas
garbanzo beans
kidney beans
lima beans
vegetarian baked beans, fat free

Canned Mexican Foods

black beans
green chiles, diced and whole
green chile enchilada sauce
red enchilada sauce
salsa, thick and chunky

Canned Asian Foods

bean sprouts
coconut milk, lite
ground fresh chili paste
soy sauce, lite
teriyaki sauce
water chestnuts, sliced

Canned Fruits/Juice

cherry filling, light
lemon juice
lime juice
mandarin oranges, in juice
pineapple chunks, in juice
pineapple, crushed, in juice

Canned Seafood

tuna, water packed
red salmon
minced clams

Frozen Foods

peas
spinach
whole-kernel corn
berries (strawberries, blueberries)
skinless, boneless chicken breasts
ground beef and/or ground turkey, 7% fat
fish portions, not breaded

Pasta, Rice, & Beans

brown rice, quick-cooking
dried black-eyed peas
dried green split peas
dried lentils
pearl barley
angel hair pasta
egg noodles (eggless)
elbow macaroni
fettucini noodles (eggless)
lasagna noodles
spaghetti noodles

Breads & Cereals

cornflake crumbs (found with the breadings)
oat bran
oatmeal
saltine crackers (unsalted tops)

Menus, Menus, Menus

J STAVER

20 Weeks of Menus—With Grocery Lists

Tips for using

The menus are really quite simple, each dinner menu consisting of a protein, starch (grain, pasta, or starchy vegetable), and a nonstarchy vegetable. Depending on your family's needs, you may also want to add an additional vegetable or another starch, such as a whole-wheat roll. Fresh fruit is also a good addition, as desserts are usually not included. A piece of fresh fruit may be just what you need to satisfy your sweet tooth. Although milk is not listed, it would be a good addition to any meal.

Most of the menu items are recipes from this cookbook. Check the recipes for the yield and adjust to meet your family's needs. You may want to double a recipe or cut it in half. When serving, adjust portion sizes to meet your individual needs.

Be sure to add to the grocery list the items that you will need for breakfast, lunch, and snacks.

Side dishes

The side dishes that are marked with an asterisk (*) are not in this cookbook. For plain vegetables, buy fresh for the best taste. Serve raw, if appropriate, or cook in the microwave (my preference) or steam. Consult your microwave cookbook for simple directions for microwaving specific vegetables.

These side dishes are on the grocery lists with a note to add the amount you need for your family for one meal. You may want to change the side dish and substitute a seasonal food, a family favorite, or a leftover. This is also a good opportunity to take advantage of foods on sale.

Amounts on grocery lists

Amounts listed on the grocery lists are the amounts needed and are not always rounded up to full containers or sizes. This way you can check what you have on hand and avoid unnecessary purchases.

Seasonings and staples

Amounts are not included on the grocery list for most seasonings and staples.

Leftovers

Take advantage of leftovers and serve within a couple of days or freeze for another time. Also freeze in individual portions for lunch. A real time-saving tip is to cook once for two meals.

You'll note that when a recipe that yields 10 or 12 servings is listed on the menu, we serve the leftovers within two days. You can instead freeze the leftovers for another week and substitute a meal of your choice.

Unfamiliar ingredients

Most ingredients are common and easily found. A few unusual items include lite coconut milk and fresh ground chili paste, which are found in the Asian section of most grocery stores. The coconut milk adds a very different flavor that is typical in Thai food and should be limited because of the saturated fat content. The chili paste is often used in very small amounts, but it stores well in the refrigerator after opening and will last for months. It is spicy-hot and can be omitted if you prefer less spicy foods. Chili paste is listed as an optional ingredient in most recipes.

Another item you may not be familiar with is hickory liquid smoke, which is often located by the barbecue sauce. This also adds another good flavor.

Menus for Weeks 19 and 20

These are great summer menus, as all recipes can be prepared without using an oven.

Abbreviations used on the Grocery Lists

tsp = teaspoon

Tbsp = tablespoon

oz = ounce

lb = pound

Dinner Menus—Week 1

Chicken in a Pocket • page 212
  5 servings

Basil Tomatoes • page 149
  4 servings

Pork Chop Suey • page 282
  4 servings
pasta of your choice*

Lemon Fish • page 261
  4 servings
broccoli*
whole-wheat roll*

Taco Soup • page 137
  6 servings
fresh orange slices*

Chicken Breasts Florentine • page 215
  6 servings
baked potato*

Week 1—Grocery List

Canned Vegetables/Sauces/Soups
(To lower sodium, choose no-added-salt or reduced-sodium products.)

cream of chicken soup, low fat, condensed (10.75 oz)
beef broth, fat free (8 oz)
chicken broth, fat free (8 oz)
bean sprouts (16 oz)
pinto or chili beans, 2 cans (15 oz each)
tomatoes, diced (28 oz)
tomato sauce (16 oz)

Pasta, Rice, & Beans
pasta of your choice*

Breads & Cereals
buttermilk biscuits (10 per 7-oz can)
whole-wheat rolls*

Fresh Produce
oranges*
lemon (4–6 slices)
green onions (4)
tomatoes (2 medium)
celery (3 stalks)
onion (2 medium)
broccoli*
baking potatoes*

Dairy & Cheese
cream cheese, fat free (8 oz)
milk, fat free (1/4 cup)
Parmesan cheese, grated (2 Tbsp)

Buy the amount for one meal or substitute a similar food.

Meat, Poultry, & Seafood
chicken breasts, skinless, boneless (2 3/4 lb)
pork tenderloin, boneless (1 lb)
fish fillets, such as snapper or sole (1 lb)
lean ground beef or ground turkey, 7% fat (1 lb)

Seasonings
salt (optional)
fresh ground pepper
dried basil
ground ginger
dried parsley
ground nutmeg
fat-free butter-flavored sprinkles

Staples
nonstick cooking spray
unbleached all-purpose flour
fresh or jar of chopped/minced garlic
molasses
lite soy sauce
cornstarch

Miscellaneous
taco seasoning (1 small package)

Frozen Foods
spinach, 2 packages (10 oz each)

Breakfast foods:

_____

_____

_____

_____

_____

Lunch foods:

_____

_____

_____

_____

_____

Snack foods:

_____

_____

_____

_____

_____

Dinner Menus—Week 2

Quick Lasagna • page 202
12 servings
tossed salad*

**Spicy Seafood and
Grapes • page 272**
4 servings
brown rice*

Leftover Quick Lasagna
tossed salad*

**Chicken Breasts in
Mushroom Sauce • page 221**
4 servings
mashed potatoes*
green beans*

Curry Tuna Salad • page 176
4 servings
Italian Focaccia Bread • page 118
12 servings

Week 2—Grocery List

Canned Vegetables/Sauces/Soups
*(To lower sodium, choose no-added-salt or
reduced-sodium products.)*
chicken broth, fat free (6 oz)
water chestnuts, sliced (8 oz)
spaghetti sauce (less than 4 g fat per
   4 oz)—32 oz

Pasta, Rice, & Beans
quick-cooking brown rice*

Canned Seafood
tuna, water packed, 2 cans (6 oz each)

Breads & Cereals
Focaccia bread, whole wheat (1 lb)

Fresh Produce
green seedless grapes (3/4 lb)
fresh ginger, minced (3 Tbsp)
broccoli florets (2 cups)
green onions (4)
mushrooms, sliced (6 oz)
lettuce leaves
salad fixings* (for two meals)
green beans*
potatoes for mashing*

Dairy & Cheese
cottage cheese, low fat (3 cups)
mozzarella cheese, reduced fat, grated,
   1 cup (4 oz)
Parmesan cheese, grated (1/3 cup)
yogurt, fat free, plain (1/2 cup)

*Buy the amount for one meal or substitute a similar food.

Meat, Poultry, & Seafood
scallops or shrimp, shelled & deveined (1 lb)
chicken breasts, skinless, boneless (1 lb)

Seasonings
salt (optional)
fresh ground pepper
dried parsley
instant chicken bouillon (to lower sodium,
    choose reduced sodium)
paprika
dried minced onion
curry powder
Italian seasoning

Staples
nonstick cooking spray
fresh or jar of chopped/minced garlic
cornstarch
granulated sugar
unbleached all-purpose flour
light mayonnaise
red wine vinegar
lite soy sauce
salad dressing (fat free or lite)

Miscellaneous
ground fresh chili paste—2 tsp (optional)—
    found in the Asian section
dry sherry (2 Tbsp)

Breakfast foods:

_____

_____

_____

_____

_____

Lunch foods:

_____

_____

_____

_____

_____

Snack foods:

_____

_____

_____

_____

_____

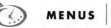

Dinner Menus—Week 3

Chicken and Broccoli Casserole • page 216
5 servings

pasta of your choice*

Spanish Baked Fish • page 264
4 servings

Roasted Root Vegetables • page 182
4 servings

Barbecued Smoked Sausage & Cabbage Casserole • page 298
5 servings

whole-grain bread*

Rolled Chicken and Asparagus • page 228
4 servings

baked sweet potato*

Meat Patties • page 290
4 servings

whole-wheat hamburger buns*
raw vegetable slices*

Week 3—Grocery List

Canned Vegetables/Sauces/Soups
(To lower sodium, choose no-added-salt or reduced-sodium products.)

mushroom pieces and stems (13.25 oz)
tomato sauce (8 oz)
cream of mushroom soup, low fat, condensed (10.75 oz)
barbecue sauce (1/3 cup)

Pasta, Rice, & Beans
pasta of your choice*

Breads & Cereals
whole-grain bread*
whole-wheat hamburger buns*
oatmeal or oat bran (1/2 cup)

Fresh Produce
broccoli florets (4 cups)
baby carrots (2 cups whole)
cabbage (1 small head)—12 oz
celery (1–2 stalks)
bell pepper, red or green (1 medium)
asparagus spears (24–30)
green onions (6)
raw vegetable slices*
onions (3 medium)
new potatoes, 4 (about 3/4 pound)
sweet potatoes*

Dairy & Cheese
milk, fat free (1/2 cup)
egg substitute (1/4 cup—equal to 1 egg)

Buy the amount for one meal or substitute a similar food.

 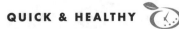

Meat, Poultry, & Seafood

chicken breasts, skinless, boneless (2 lb)
fish fillets, such as snapper or sole (1 lb)
turkey smoked sausage, low fat (1 lb)
lean ground beef or ground turkey,
    7% fat (1 lb)

Seasonings

salt (optional)
fresh ground pepper
dried rosemary
paprika
chili powder
dried oregano
ground cumin
dried thyme
dried parsley
ground mustard

Staples

nonstick cooking spray
lemon juice
fresh or jar of chopped/minced garlic
olive oil

Breakfast foods:

_____

_____

_____

_____

_____

Lunch foods:

_____

_____

_____

_____

_____

Snack foods:

_____

_____

_____

_____

_____

Dinner Menus—Week 4

Sweet and Sour Chicken • page 244
5 servings

brown rice*

**Grilled Salmon with
Corn Salsa** • page 252
8 servings

sliced new potatoes* (cover and bake or
microwave)—a favorite is Yukon gold

Three-Bean Soup • page 140
12 servings

low-fat cottage cheese on lettuce leaf*

**Hickory-Smoked Barbecued
Chicken** • page 241
4 servings

whole-wheat roll*

Roasted Eggplant Medley
(make 1/2 recipe) • page 147
4 servings

Leftover Three-Bean Soup

Lime Cottage Salad • page 160
7 servings

Week 4—Grocery List

Canned Fruits & Juices
pineapple chunks, in juice (8 oz)
pineapple, crushed, in juice (20 oz)

Canned Vegetables/Sauces/Soups
*(To lower sodium, choose no-added-salt or
reduced-sodium products.)*

kidney beans (15 oz)
black-eyed peas (15 oz)
garbanzo beans (15 oz)
tomatoes, diced (14.5 oz)
tomatoes, diced (28 oz)
tomato paste (6 oz)
chicken broth, fat free (10 oz)

Pasta, Rice, & Beans
quick-cooking brown rice*

Breads & Cereals
whole-wheat rolls*
cottage cheese, low-fat*

Fresh Produce
celery (2 stalks)
bell peppers: green, red, or yellow (3)
cucumber (1/2 medium)
fresh cilantro, chopped (1/4 cup)
carrots (2)
zucchini (1 small) or celery (2 stalks)
eggplant, 1 small (about 6–7 oz)
tomatoes (1 medium)
6–10 lettuce leaves*
onion (2 medium)
new potatoes*

Dairy & Cheese
yogurt, fat free, plain (1 cup)
cottage cheese, low fat (2 cups)

*Buy the amount for one meal or substitute a similar food.

 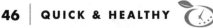

Meat, Poultry, & Seafood
salmon fillets (2 lb)
chicken breasts, skinless, boneless (2 lb)
*(Note: This is for 2 recipes. For 1 recipe,
you can substitute 2 lb chicken parts for
1 lb of skinless, boneless chicken breasts.)*

Seasonings
salt (optional)
fresh ground pepper
garlic powder
cayenne pepper
chili powder
dried basil
dried oregano
ground cumin
ground ginger
Italian seasoning

Staples
nonstick cooking spray
fresh or jar of chopped/minced garlic
cider vinegar
lite soy sauce
brown sugar
cornstarch
red wine vinegar
Dijon mustard
hickory liquid smoke (found by the
    barbecue sauce)

Miscellaneous
lime-flavored gelatin, sugar free (0.3 oz)

Frozen Foods
whole-kernel corn (2 cups)
whipped topping, fat free (6 oz)

Breakfast foods:

_____

_____

_____

_____

_____

Lunch foods:

_____

_____

_____

_____

_____

Snack foods:

_____

_____

_____

_____

_____

Dinner Menus—Week 5

Chicken Enchiladas • page 235
8 servings

tossed salad*

Meat Loaf • page 296
6 servings

steamed red potatoes* (cover and bake or microwave)

Baked Portobello Mushrooms • page 146
4 servings

Pork and Rice Casserole • page 280
4 servings

spinach*

Thai Chicken Soup • page 135
6 servings

fresh fruit slices*

Sweet Mustard Fish • page 266
4 servings

whole-wheat roll*

Pear Salad with Raspberry Dressing • page 157
5 servings

Week 5—Grocery List

Canned Vegetables/Sauces/Soups
(To lower sodium, choose no-added-salt or reduced-sodium products.)

cream of celery soup, low fat, condensed (10.75 oz)
chicken broth, fat free (32 oz)
salsa, thick and chunky (1/2 cup)
enchilada sauce, 2 cans (10 oz each)

Pasta, Rice, & Beans
quick-cooking brown rice (1 cup)
angel hair pasta (6 oz)

Breads & Cereals
corn tortillas (6-inch)—12
whole-wheat rolls*

Fresh Produce
pears (2)
fruit*
green bell pepper (1 small)
red bell pepper (2 medium)
celery (1–2 stalks)
broccoli florets (2 cups)
snow pea pods (2 cups)
fresh ginger, minced (2 Tbsp)
salad greens, 10–12 oz (about 2 quarts) plus salad fixings*
spinach*
onion (3 medium)
red potatoes*

Dairy & Cheese
cottage cheese or Ricotta cheese, low fat (1 cup)
yogurt, fat free, plain (1 cup)
cheddar or Mexican blend cheese, reduced fat, grated, 1/2 cup (2 oz)

Buy the amount for one meal or substitute a similar food.

mozzarella cheese, reduced fat, grated, 1/2 cup (2 oz)
milk, fat free (3/4 cup)
egg substitute (1/4 cup—equal to 1 egg)

Meat, Poultry, & Seafood
chicken breasts, skinless, boneless (2 lb)
pork top loin, boneless (1 lb)
fish fillets, such as snapper or sole (1 lb)
lean ground beef or ground turkey, 7% fat (1 1/2 lb)

Seasonings
salt (optional)
fresh ground pepper
dried parsley
ground mustard
dried rosemary
dried marjoram
dried thyme
ground cumin

Staples
nonstick cooking spray
fresh or jar of chopped/minced garlic
olive oil
lite soy sauce
Dijon mustard
honey (2 Tbsp)
lemon juice
salad dressing (fat-free or lite)

Miscellaneous
walnuts (1/4 cup chopped)
raspberry salad dressing, reduced fat (1/2 cup)
ground fresh chili paste—1 Tbsp (optional)— found in the Asian section

Breakfast foods:

_____

_____

_____

_____

_____

Lunch foods:

_____

_____

_____

_____

_____

Snack foods:

_____

_____

_____

_____

_____

Dinner Menus—Week 6

Chicken Breasts Supreme • page 244
8 servings
mashed potatoes*
carrots*

**New England Fish
Chowder • page 134**
4 servings
Greek Salad • page 164
8 servings - (use leftovers with Sloppy Joes)

Sloppy Joes • page 200
5 servings
tossed salad* (or leftover Greek Salad)

**Mexican-Style Chicken
and Rice • page 238**
5 servings
whole-wheat tortillas*

Oven-Fried Pork Loin • page 278
4 servings
baked sweet potato*
**Zucchini, Tomato,
and Onion • page 148**
7 servings

Week 6—Grocery List

Canned Vegetables/Sauces/Soups
*(To lower sodium, choose no-added-salt or
reduced-sodium products.)*
chicken broth, fat free (4 oz)
tomato soup, condensed (10.75 oz)
tomatoes, diced (14.5 oz)
green chiles, diced (4 oz)

Pasta, Rice, & Beans
quick-cooking brown rice (1 cup)

Breads & Cereals
cornflake crumbs (3/4 cup)—found
    with the breadings
whole-grain hamburger buns (2 oz each)—5
whole-wheat tortillas*

Fresh Produce
mushrooms, sliced (6 oz)
tomatoes (2 medium)
zucchini (2 small)
cucumber (1 medium)
onions (4 medium)
green bell peppers (3 medium)
red bell pepper (1 medium)
yellow bell pepper (1 medium)
carrots*
salad fixings*—or leftover Greek Salad
sweet potatoes*
white potatoes (1/2 lb)
potatoes for mashing*

Dairy & Cheese
milk, fat free (2 cups)
feta cheese, fat free (4 oz)
cheddar cheese or Mexican cheese,
    reduced fat, grated, 1/2 cup (2 oz)

*Buy the amount for one meal or substitute a similar food.

 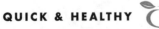

Meat, Poultry, & Seafood
chicken breasts, skinless, boneless (3 lb)
fish fillets (12 oz)
scallops, fish can be substituted (4 oz)
lean ground beef or ground turkey,
    7% fat (1 lb)
boneless top loin pork chops, about
    3/4-inch to 1-inch thick (1 lb)

Seasonings
salt (optional)
fresh ground pepper
dried thyme
dried sage
dried oregano
ground cumin
Italian seasoning

Staples
nonstick cooking spray
cornstarch
prepared mustard
red wine vinegar
lemon juice
fresh or jar of chopped/minced garlic
Tabasco sauce
salad dressing (fat free or lite)

Miscellaneous
dry white wine, vermouth, or chicken
    broth (1/2 cup)

Breakfast foods:
_____

_____

_____

_____

_____

Lunch foods:
_____

_____

_____

_____

_____

Snack foods:
_____

_____

_____

_____

_____

Dinner Menus—Week 7

Chicken and Biscuits • page 218
5 servings
raw vegetable slices*

Chinese Pepper Steak • page 281
4 servings
brown rice*

**Grilled Salmon with
Fruit Salsa • page 254**
4 servings
asparagus*
whole-grain bread*

French Glazed Chicken • page 227
4 servings
Brussels sprouts*

**Cheese-Stuffed Potatoes
(make 1/2 recipe) • page 183**
4 servings

John Torrey • page 302
6 servings
tossed salad*

Week 7—Grocery List

Canned Vegetables/Sauces/Soups
(To lower sodium, choose no-added-salt or reduced-sodium products.)

beef broth, fat free (2 cups)
chicken broth, fat free (2 3/4 cups)
tomatoes, diced (14.5 oz)
tomato sauce (8 oz)
artichoke hearts, quartered (14 oz)
chopped pimiento (2 oz)
mushroom pieces and stems (4 oz)

Pasta, Rice, & Beans
elbow macaroni (6 oz)
quick-cooking brown rice*

Breads & Cereals
buttermilk biscuits (10 per can)—7 oz
whole-grain bread*

Fresh Produce
fresh fruit, such as red papaya, nectarine,
    apricot, or peaches—2 cups cubed
mushrooms, sliced (8 oz)
celery (2 stalks)
avocado (1 medium)
green onions (3)
green bell pepper (3 medium)
asparagus*
Brussels sprouts*
raw vegetable slices*
salad fixings*
potatoes, 2 (about 5 oz each)
onion (2 medium)

*Buy the amount for one meal or substitute a similar food.

 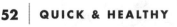

Dairy & Cheese
cottage cheese, low fat (1/2 cup)
milk, fat free (1 tablespoon)
cheddar cheese, reduced fat, grated,
   3/4 cup (3 oz)

Meat, Poultry, & Seafood
chicken breasts, skinless, boneless (2 lb)
beef top sirloin, boneless (1 lb)
salmon fillets (1 lb)
lean ground beef or ground turkey,
   7% fat (1 lb)

Seasonings
salt (optional)
fresh ground pepper
dried parsley
dried minced onion
paprika
chili powder

Staples
nonstick cooking spray
unbleached all-purpose flour
fresh or jar of chopped/minced garlic
lite soy sauce
cornstarch
granulated sugar
lime juice
salad dressing (fat-free or lite)

Miscellaneous
French dressing, fat free (1/4 cup)
apricot preserves, sugar free (2 Tbsp)

Frozen Foods
peas or corn (1 cup)

Breakfast foods:

_____

_____

_____

_____

_____

Lunch foods:

_____

_____

_____

_____

_____

Snack foods:

_____

_____

_____

_____

_____

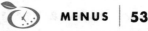

Dinner Menus—Week 8

Chicken and Artichokes Dijon • page 219
4 servings
fresh fruit slices*

Swedish Meatballs (20 meatballs) • page 293
4 servings
mashed potatoes*
broccoli*

Minestrone Soup • page 139
10 servings
Lime Cottage Salad • page 160
7 servings

Polynesian Fish • page 257
4 servings
pasta of your choice*
Romaine and Mandarin Orange Salad • page 161
5 servings

Leftover Minestrone Soup
low-fat cottage cheese on lettuce leaf*

Week 8—Grocery List

Canned Fruits & Juices
pineapple, crushed, in juice (20 oz)
mandarin oranges, 2 cans, in juice (11 oz each)

Canned Vegetables/Sauces/Soups
(To lower sodium, choose no-added-salt or reduced-sodium products.)

beef or chicken broth, fat free (44 oz)
chicken broth, fat free (2 oz)
tomatoes, diced (14 oz)

Pasta, Rice, & Beans
quick-cooking brown rice (1 cup)
dried green split peas (1/3 cup)
dried lentils (1/3 cup)
pearl barley (1/3 cup)
dried black-eyed peas (1/2 cup)
pasta of your choice*

Breads & Cereals
oatmeal or oat bran, 1 cup**

Fresh Produce
fruit*
red bell pepper (1 medium)
vegetables (celery, onion, zucchini, carrots, green pepper, mushrooms), 2 1/2 cups chopped
avocado (1 medium)
salad greens, 10–12 oz (about 2 quarts)
broccoli*
6–10 lettuce leaves*
potatoes for mashing*

Dairy & Cheese
yogurt, fat free, plain (1 1/4 cups)
milk, fat free (1 cup)**
egg substitute (1/2 cup)—equal to 2 eggs**
Parmesan cheese, grated (3 Tbsp)

Buy the amount for one meal or substitute a similar food.

 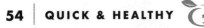

cottage cheese, low fat (2 cups plus
    enough for one side dish)

Meat, Poultry, & Seafood
chicken breasts, skinless, boneless (1 lb)
lean ground beef or ground turkey,
    7% fat (2 lb)**
firm fish, such as salmon or snapper (1 lb)

Seasonings
salt (optional)
fresh ground pepper
dried parsley
onion powder**
ground nutmeg**
dried basil
dried oregano
bay leaves
ground ginger
ground mustard

Staples
nonstick cooking spray
light mayonnaise
Dijon mustard
granulated sugar
fresh or jar of chopped/minced garlic
unbleached all-purpose flour
brown sugar
lite soy sauce
hickory liquid smoke (found by the
    barbecue sauce)
lime juice
rice vinegar
canola oil

Miscellaneous
lime-flavored gelatin, sugar free (0.3 oz)

Frozen
whipped topping, fat free (6 oz)

**If using leftover frozen meatballs, omit these ingredients.

Breakfast foods:

_____

_____

_____

_____

_____

Lunch foods:

_____

_____

_____

_____

_____

Snack foods:

_____

_____

_____

_____

_____

Dinner Menus—Week 9

Teriyaki Chicken Stir-Fry • page 247
  4 servings
brown rice*

Orange Pork Chops • page 279
  4 servings
baked potato*
zucchini*

Poached Fish • page 265
  4 servings
corn*
Basil Tomatoes • page 149
  4 servings

Moore • page 303
  4 servings
tossed salad*

Tortilla Soup • page 143
  4 servings
fresh fruit*

Week 9—Grocery List

Canned Vegetables/Sauces/Soups
(To lower sodium, choose no-added-salt or reduced-sodium products.)

chicken broth, fat free (36 oz)
tomato soup, condensed (10.75 oz)
tomatoes, diced (14.5 oz)
black beans (15 oz)
green chiles, diced (4 oz)
teriyaki sauce (1/4 cup)

Pasta, Rice, & Beans
fettuccini noodles (eggless)—6 oz
quick-cooking brown rice*

Breads & Cereals
3 corn tortillas

Fresh Produce
fresh fruit*
red bell pepper (1 medium)
green bell pepper (1 medium)
tomatoes (2 medium)
green onions (5–6 bunches)
zucchini*
salad fixings*
baking potatoes*

Dairy & Cheese
cheddar cheese, reduced fat, grated,
  1/4 cup (1 oz)

Meat, Poultry, & Seafood
chicken breasts, skinless, boneless (1 1/2 lb)
4 pork rib chops, with bone (cut 3 per lb)
fish fillets, such as snapper or sole (1 lb)
lean ground beef or ground turkey,
  7% fat (1 lb)

Buy the amount for one meal or substitute a similar food.

 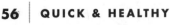

Seasonings
salt (optional)
fresh ground pepper
bay leaves
dried basil

Staples
nonstick cooking spray
fresh or jar of chopped/minced garlic
Dijon mustard
lemon juice
salad dressing (fat free or lite)

Miscellaneous
dry-roasted peanuts, unsalted (1/3 cup)
sugar-free or low-sugar orange
    marmalade (1/3 cup)

Frozen Foods
whole-kernel corn (1 1/3 cups plus enough
    for one side dish)

Breakfast foods: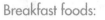

_____

_____

_____

_____

_____

Lunch foods:

_____

_____

_____

_____

_____

Snack foods:

_____

_____

_____

_____

_____

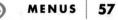

Dinner Menus—Week 10

Tortilla Pie • page 301
10 servings
Grapefruit and Avocado Salad • page 156
5 servings

Yogurt Cumin Fish • page 268
4 servings
sliced new potatoes* (cover and bake or microwave)—a favorite is Yukon gold
Marinated Vegetables • page 152
8 servings

Leftover Tortilla Pie
Leftover Marinated Vegetables

Pork Stir-Fry • page 286
4 servings
whole-wheat pita bread*

Chicken Cacciatore • page 246
6 servings
pasta of your choice*
fresh fruit slices*

Week 10—Grocery List

Canned Vegetables/Sauces/Soups
(To lower sodium, choose no-added-salt or reduced-sodium products.)

stewed tomatoes (14 oz)
tomato sauce (16 oz)
thick and chunky salsa (2 cups)
creamed corn (15 oz)

Pasta, Rice, & Beans
pasta of your choice*

Breads & Cereals
corn tortillas (6-inch)—12
whole-wheat pita bread*

Fresh Produce
grapefruit (1)
fruit*
avocado (1 medium)
green onions (2)
salad greens, 10–12 oz (about 2 quarts)
onion (1 medium and 2 large)
broccoli florets (2 cups)
carrots (2)
red bell pepper (1 medium)
zucchini (1 small)
vegetables, such as: broccoli, celery, green pepper, carrots, mushrooms, cauliflower, green beans (4 cups)
new potatoes*

Dairy & Cheese
yogurt, fat-free plain (1/3 cup)
cheddar cheese or Mexican blend cheese, reduced-fat, grated, 3/4 cup (3 oz)

Buy the amount for one meal or substitute a similar food.

 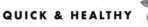

Meat, Poultry, & Seafood
chicken breasts, skinless, boneless (1 1/2 lb)
fish fillets, such as snapper or sole (1 lb)
pork tenderloin (1 lb)
lean ground beef or ground turkey,
   7% fat (2 lb)

Seasonings
salt (optional)
fresh ground pepper
chili powder
garlic powder
ground cumin
Italian seasoning

Staples
nonstick cooking spray
lime juice
apple cider vinegar
olive oil
granulated sugar
fresh or jar of chopped/minced garlic
lite soy sauce

Miscellaneous
apricot preserves, sugar free (3 Tbsp)
Italian dressing, reduced fat (1/4 cup)

Frozen Foods
peas (2 cups)

Breakfast foods:
_____
_____
_____
_____
_____

Lunch foods:
_____
_____
_____
_____
_____

Snack foods:
_____
_____
_____
_____

Dinner Menus—Week 11

Chicken Nuggets • page 223
4 servings
cauliflower*
Sweet Potato Fries • page 186
4 servings

Quick Meat Lasagna • page 297
12 servings
tossed salad*

French Glazed Fish • page 262
4 servings
whole-wheat roll*
green beans*

Leftover Quick Meat Lasagna
tossed salad*

Chicken and Pea Pod Stir-Fry • page 242
4 servings
brown rice*

Week 11—Grocery List

Canned Vegetables/Sauces/Soups
spaghetti sauce (less than 4 g fat per 4 oz)—32 oz

Pasta, Rice, & Beans
lasagna noodles (3/4 lb)
quick-cooking brown rice*

Breads & Cereals
cornflake crumbs (1/2 cup)—found with the breadings
whole-wheat rolls*

Fresh Produce
carrots (3)
fresh snow pea pods (2 cups)
green onions (4)
cauliflower*
salad fixings* (for two meals)
green beans*
sweet potatoes, 4 medium (about 4 oz each)

Dairy & Cheese
cottage cheese or Ricotta cheese, low fat (2 cups)
mozzarella cheese, reduced fat, grated, 1 cup (4 oz)
Parmesan cheese, grated (1/4 cup)

Meat, Poultry, & Seafood
chicken breasts, skinless, boneless (2 lb)
lean ground beef or ground turkey, 7% fat (1 lb)
fish fillets, such as snapper or sole (1 lb)

Buy the amount for one meal or substitute a similar food.

 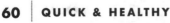

Seasonings
salt (optional)
fresh ground pepper
dried thyme
dried sage
anise seed
fennel seed
dried parsley
dried minced onion

Staples
nonstick cooking spray
fresh or jar of chopped/minced garlic
lite soy sauce
cornstarch
canola oil
salad dressing (fat free or lite)

Miscellaneous
French dressing, fat free (1/4 cup)
apricot preserves, sugar free (2 Tbsp)

Breakfast foods:

_____

_____

_____

_____

_____

Lunch foods:

_____

_____

_____

_____

_____

Snack foods:

_____

_____

_____

_____

_____

Dinner Menus—Week 12

Fillets of Sole Thermidor • page 269
8 servings
asparagus*
baked potato*

Chicken Tortilla Casserole • page 233
10 servings
Salsa Vegetables • page 153
8 servings

Meatball Sandwich/ 16 meatballs • page 196
4 servings
Gourmet Cucumbers • page 151
6 servings

Leftover Chicken Tortilla Casserole
sliced tomatoes*

Mandarin Orange Seafood • page 273
4 servings
pasta of your choice*

Week 12—Grocery List

Canned Fruits & Juices
mandarin oranges, in juice (10.5 oz)

Canned Vegetables/Sauces/Soups
(To lower sodium, choose no-added-salt or reduced-sodium products.)

cream of chicken soup, low fat, condensed—
   2 cans (10.75 oz each)
chicken broth, fat free (6 oz)
green chiles, diced (7 oz)
water chestnuts, sliced (8 oz)
tomatoes, diced (14.5 oz)
spaghetti sauce (less than 4 g fat per
   4 oz)—8 oz

Pasta, Rice, & Beans
pasta of your choice*

Breads & Cereals
whole-grain rolls (2 oz each)—4
oatmeal or oat bran, 1 cup**

Fresh Produce
cucumber (2 medium)
red bell pepper (2 1/2 medium)
fresh cilantro, chopped (1/4 cup)
sweet onion (1 medium)
fresh ginger, minced (1 Tbsp)
green onions (4)
asparagus*
sliced tomatoes*
baking potatoes*

Dairy & Cheese
milk, fat free (1 3/4 cups)**
egg substitute (1/2 cup)—equal to 2 eggs**
cheddar cheese, reduced fat, grated,
   1 cup (4 oz)

*Buy the amount for one meal or substitute a similar food.

Meat, Poultry, & Seafood
fillets of sole (2 lb)
chicken breasts, skinless, boneless (1 3/4 lb)
lean ground beef or ground turkey,
   7% fat (2 lb)**
scallops or shrimp (shelled & deveined) (1 lb)

Seasonings
salt (optional)
fresh ground pepper
fat-free butter-flavored sprinkles
dash of paprika
dried minced onion
ground cumin
garlic powder
cayenne pepper
onion powder**
dried parsley**
ground nutmeg**

Staples
nonstick cooking spray
rice vinegar
red wine vinegar
cornstarch
granulated sugar
lite soy sauce

Frozen Foods
whole-kernel corn (2/3 cup)

Breakfast foods:
_____
_____
_____
_____

Lunch foods:
_____
_____
_____
_____
_____

Snack foods:
_____
_____
_____
_____
_____

**If using leftover frozen meatballs, omit these ingredients.*

Dinner Menus—Week 13

Polynesian Chicken • page 213
4 servings
brown rice*
**Pear Salad with
Raspberry Dressing • page 157**
5 servings

Chili Con Carne • page 142
12 servings
sliced cucumbers*

Mediterranean Seafood • page 270
4 servings
whole-grain bread*

Baked Chimichangas • page 232
4 servings
Mexican Garden Salad • page 162
4 servings

Leftover Chili Con Carne
fresh fruit slices*

Week 13—Grocery List

Canned Vegetables/Sauces/Soups
(To lower sodium, choose no-added-salt or reduced-sodium products.)

chicken broth, fat free (6 oz)
kidney beans, 3 cans (15 oz, each)
tomatoes, diced (28 oz)
tomato sauce (16 oz)
salsa, thick and chunky (3/4 cup)

Pasta, Rice, & Beans
pasta of your choice (4 oz)
quick-cooking brown rice*

Breads & Cereals
whole-wheat tortillas (8 inch)—4
whole-grain bread*

Fresh Produce
pears (2 medium)
fruit*
salad greens, 10–12 oz (about 2 quarts)
mushrooms, sliced (8 oz)
broccoli florets (2 cups)
green onions (2)
tomato (1 medium)
cucumber (1/2 medium), plus slices for one
    side dish
avocado (1 medium)
fresh cilantro, chopped (1/2 cup)
red bell pepper (2 medium)
green peppers (2 medium)
onions, medium (1 sweet and 2 yellow)

Dairy & Cheese
cheddar or Mexican blend cheese,
    reduced fat, grated, 1/2 cup (2 oz)

Buy the amount for one meal or substitute a similar food.

 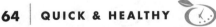

Meat, Poultry, & Seafood

chicken breasts, skinless, boneless (1 3/4 lb)
*(Note: This is for 2 recipes. For 1 recipe,
you can substitute 2 lb chicken parts for
1 lb of skinless, boneless chicken breasts.)*
lean ground beef or ground turkey,
7% fat (2 lb)
scallops or cleaned shrimp (1 lb)

Seasonings

salt (optional)
fresh ground pepper
ground ginger
ground mustard
chili powder
paprika
bay leaves
Italian seasoning
ground cumin

Staples

nonstick cooking spray
brown sugar
fresh or jar of chopped/minced garlic
lime juice
lemon juice
lite soy sauce
hickory liquid smoke (found by the
barbecue sauce)

Miscellaneous

raspberry salad dressing, reduced fat
(1/2 cup)
walnuts (1/4 cup chopped)

Breakfast foods:

_____

_____

_____

_____

_____

Lunch foods:

_____

_____

_____

_____

_____

Snack foods:

_____

_____

_____

_____

_____

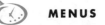

Dinner Menus—Week 14

Crispy Potato Chicken • page 225
4 servings

Roasted Eggplant Medley
(make 1/2 recipe) • page 147
4 servings

Spaghetti and Meatballs
(24 meatballs) • page 292
6 servings

tossed salad*

**Hickory-Smoked
Barbecued Fish** • page 256
4 servings

broccoli*

Herb Potato Salad • page 170
6 servings

**Spicy Chicken and
Grapes** • page 243
5 servings

whole-wheat roll*

Crusty Calzone
(ground meat filling) • page 194
8 servings

raw vegetable slices*

Week 14—Grocery List

Canned Vegetables/Sauces/Soups
*(To lower sodium, choose no-added-salt or
reduced-sodium products.)*

spaghetti sauce (less than 4 g fat per
    4 oz)—26 oz
pizza sauce (1/4 cup)
chicken broth, fat free (8 oz)

Pasta, Rice, & Beans
spaghetti noodles (3 1/2 oz)

Breads & Cereals
oatmeal or oat bran, 1 cup**
whole-wheat rolls*

Fresh Produce
green seedless grapes (3/4 lb)
eggplant, 1 small (about 6–7 oz)
onion (1 medium)
green pepper (1 medium)
tomatoes (1 medium)
celery (2 stalks)
green onions (2)
fresh ginger, minced (3 Tbsp)
broccoli florets (2 cups plus enough
    for one side dish)
salad fixings*
raw vegetable slices*
new potatoes (1 1/2 lb)

Dairy & Cheese
milk, fat free (1 cup)**
egg substitute (1/2 cup)—equal to 2 eggs**
yogurt, fat free, plain (3 tablespoons)
mozzarella cheese, reduced fat, grated,
    1 cup (4 oz)

Buy the amount for one meal or substitute a similar food.

 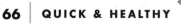

Meat, Poultry, & Seafood
chicken breasts, skinless, boneless (2 lb)
lean ground beef or ground turkey,
    7% fat (2 1/2 lb)**
firm fish, such as salmon, snapper,
    or halibut (1 lb)

Seasonings
salt (optional)
fresh ground pepper
Italian seasoning
dried parsley**
ground nutmeg**
ground ginger
dried basil
dried thyme
onion powder
garlic powder

Staples
nonstick cooking spray
Dijon mustard
fresh or jar of chopped/minced garlic
lemon juice
canola oil
lite soy sauce
hickory liquid smoke (found by the
    barbecue sauce)
light mayonnaise
cornstarch
granulated sugar
red wine vinegar
salad dressing (fat free or lite)

Frozen Foods
whole-wheat bread dough—1 lb

Miscellaneous
ground fresh chili paste—2 tsp (optional)—
    found in the Asian section

**If using leftover frozen meatballs, omit these ingredients.*

Breakfast foods:

_____

_____

_____

_____

_____

Lunch foods:

_____

_____

_____

_____

_____

Snack foods:

_____

_____

_____

_____

_____

Dinner Menus—Week 15

Mandarin Orange Chicken • page 245
4 servings

brown rice*

Asparagus Topped Meatloaf • page 294
4 servings

baked sweet potato*

Sausage and Bean Soup • page 141
8 servings

fresh fruit slices*

Mediterranean Chicken • page 214
6 servings

whole-wheat roll*

Oven-Fried Fish • page 259
4 servings

sliced tomatoes and cucumbers*

Low-Fat French Fries • page 185
4 servings

Week 15—Grocery List

Canned Fruits & Juices
mandarin oranges, in juice (10.5 oz)

Canned Vegetables/Sauces/Soups
(To lower sodium, choose no-added-salt or reduced-sodium products.)

chicken broth, fat free (24 oz)
cream of mushroom soup, low fat, condensed (10.75 oz)
beans of your choosing (black, kidney, pinto, garbanzo, lima), 4 cans (15 oz each)
tomatoes, diced (14.5 oz)
mushroom pieces and stems (13.25 oz)
water chestnuts, sliced (8 oz)
salsa, thick and chunky (1/2 cup)
green chiles, diced (4 oz)

Pasta, Rice, & Beans
pasta of your choice (6 oz)
quick-cooking brown rice*

Breads & Cereals
oatmeal or oat bran (1/2 cup)
cornflake crumbs (1/4 cup)—found with the breadings
whole-wheat rolls*

*Buy the amount for one meal or substitute a similar food.

Fresh Produce
fruit*
fresh ginger, minced (1 Tbsp)
red bell pepper (4 medium)
green onions (4)
asparagus (3/4 lb)
onion (1 medium)
potatoes, 4 medium (about 5 oz each)
sweet potatoes*
mushrooms, sliced (8 oz)
broccoli florets (2 cups)
sliced tomatoes and cucumbers*

Dairy & Cheese
milk, fat free (1/4 cup)
egg substitute (1/4 cup—equal to 1 egg)

Meat, Poultry, & Seafood
chicken breasts, skinless, boneless (2 lb)
turkey smoked sausage, low fat (1 lb)
lean ground beef or ground turkey,
    7% fat (1 lb)
fish fillets, such as snapper, sole,
    or halibut (1 lb)

Seasonings
salt (optional)
fresh ground pepper
dried parsley
paprika
Italian seasoning
crushed red pepper

Staples
nonstick cooking spray
cornstarch
canola oil
lite soy sauce

Breakfast foods:

_____

_____

_____

_____

_____

Lunch foods:

_____

_____

_____

_____

_____

Snack foods:

_____

_____

_____

_____

_____

Dinner Menus—Week 16

Pizza Meat Loaf • page 295
4 servings
whole-kernel corn*
raw or cooked baby carrots*

Chicken and Vegetables in Gravy • page 217
6 servings
mashed potatoes*

Beef or Pork Fajitas • page 283
4 servings
orange slices*

Italian Broccoli and Pasta • page 204
4 servings
low-fat cottage cheese on lettuce leaf*

Yogurt Cumin Chicken • page 226
4 servings
whole-wheat roll*
Brussels sprouts*

Week 16—Grocery List

Canned Vegetables/Sauces/Soups
(To lower sodium, choose no-added-salt or reduced-sodium products.)

chicken broth, fat free (12 oz)
artichoke hearts, quartered (14 oz)
mushroom pieces and stems (13.25 oz)
tomatoes, stewed (14 oz)
pizza sauce (1/4 cup)

Pasta, Rice, & Beans
fettucini noodles, eggless (2 1/2 oz)

Breads & Cereals
whole-wheat tortillas, 4 (8-inch) or 8 (6-inch)
whole-wheat rolls*

Fresh Produce
oranges*
vegetables thin sliced (1/2 cup, such as
    green pepper and onion)
green bell pepper (1 medium)
onion (1 medium)
broccoli florets (2 cups)
green onion (1)
baby carrots*
6–10 lettuce leaves*
Brussels sprouts*
potatoes for mashing*

Dairy & Cheese
mozzarella cheese, reduced fat, grated,
    1/4 cup (1 oz)—optional
Parmesan cheese, grated (2 tsp)
yogurt, fat free, plain (1/3 cup)
cottage cheese, low fat*

Buy the amount for one meal or substitute a similar food.

 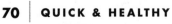

Meat, Poultry, & Seafood
top sirloin or pork tenderloin, boneless (1 lb)
lean ground beef or ground turkey,
    7% fat (1 lb)
chicken breasts, skinless, boneless (2 1/2 lb)
    *(Note: This is for 2 recipes. For 1 recipe,
    you can substitute 2 1/2–3 lb chicken parts for
    1 1/2 lb of skinless, boneless chicken breasts.)*

Seasonings
salt (optional)
fresh ground pepper
paprika
dried rosemary
dried cilantro
chili powder
dried thyme
dried oregano
ground cumin

Staples
nonstick cooking spray
unbleached all-purpose flour

Miscellaneous
dry sherry or fat-free chicken broth (3 oz)
apricot preserves, sugar free (3 Tbsp)

Frozen
whole-kernel corn*

Breakfast foods:
_____
_____
_____
_____
_____

Lunch foods:
_____
_____
_____
_____
_____

Snack foods:
_____
_____
_____
_____
_____

Dinner Menus—Week 17

Tortilla Pie • page 301
10 servings
raw vegetable slices*

Chicken Curry Soup • page 138
4 servings
tossed salad*

Leftover Tortilla Pie
raw vegetable slices*

Salmon Cakes • page 258
4 servings
whole-wheat hamburger buns
lettuce and tomato slices*

Creamy Cabbage
Stir-fry • page 300
4 servings
fresh fruit*

Week 17—Grocery List

Canned Vegetables/Sauces/Soups
(To lower sodium, choose no-added-salt or reduced-sodium products.)

thick and chunky salsa (2 cups)
tomato sauce (8 oz)
creamed corn (15 oz)
chicken broth, fat free (32 oz)
cream of celery soup, low fat,
   condensed (10.75 oz)

Canned Seafood
red salmon (15 oz)

Pasta, Rice, & Beans
quick-cooking brown rice (2/3 cup)
egg noodles, eggless (4 oz)

Breads & Cereals
whole-wheat hamburger buns
   (2 oz each)—4
corn tortillas (6-inch)—12
saltines—6 (unsalted top)

Fresh Produce
apple (1 medium)
fresh fruit*
onion (4 large)
red bell pepper (1 small)
cabbage (1 small head)—12 oz
lettuce and tomato slices*
salad fixings*
vegetable slices* (for two meals)

*Buy the amount for one meal or substitute a similar food.

 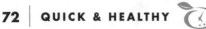

Dairy & Cheese

cheddar cheese or Mexican blend cheese,
  reduced fat, grated, 3/4 cups (4 oz)

Meat, Poultry, & Seafood

lean ground beef or ground turkey,
  7% fat (2 lb)
chicken breasts, skinless, boneless (1 lb)
lean ground turkey or beef, 7% fat (1 lb)

Seasonings

salt (optional)
fresh ground pepper
ground cumin
garlic powder
chili powder
curry powder
onion powder

Staples

nonstick cooking spray
unbleached all-purpose flour
Miracle Whip Light
lemon juice
Tabasco sauce
salad dressing (fat free or lite)

Breakfast foods:

_____

_____

_____

_____

_____

Lunch foods:

_____

_____

_____

_____

_____

Snack foods:

_____

_____

_____

_____

_____

Dinner Menus—Week 18

Turkey French Dips • page 192
4 servings

raw carrot slices*

Italian Cioppino • page 133
4 servings

whole-grain bread*

Oven-Fried Chicken • page 222
6 servings

Sweet Potato Fries • page 186
4 servings

Gourmet Cucumbers • page 151
6 servings

Piled-High Vegetable Pizza • page 198
6 servings

tossed salad*

Green Chile Chicken Enchilada Casserole • page 234
8 servings

fresh orange and grapefruit sections*

Week 18—Grocery List

Canned Vegetables/Sauces/Soups
(To lower sodium, choose no-added-salt or reduced-sodium products.)

green chile enchilada sauce (28 oz)
green chiles, diced (7 oz)
tomatoes, diced (28 oz)
tomato sauce (8 oz)
pizza sauce (1/2 cup)
chicken broth, fat-free or white wine (4 oz)

Breads & Cereals
whole-grain rolls (2 oz each)—4
cornflake crumbs (1/4 cup)—found
    with the breadings
thin pizza crust (such as Boboli)—1 (10 oz)
corn tortillas (6-inch)—12
whole-grain bread*

Fresh Produce
oranges and grapefruit*
bell pepper, green or yellow (1 medium)
tomatoes (2 medium)
cucumber (1 medium)
eggplant, 1 small (about 12–14 oz)
raw carrot slices*
salad fixings*
onions, medium (1 sweet and 2 yellow)
sweet potatoes, 4 medium (about 4 oz each)

Dairy & Cheese
mozzarella cheese, reduced fat, grated,
    1 1/2 cups (6 oz)
cheddar or Mexican cheese, reduced fat,
    grated, 1 cup (4 oz)
sour cream, fat free (1/2 cup)

Buy the amount for one meal or substitute a similar food.

Meat, Poultry & Seafood

turkey slices, cooked (8 oz)
fish fillets or cleaned shrimp, clams,
    or crab (1 lb)
chicken breasts, skinless, boneless (3 1/4 lb)
    (Note: This is for 2 recipes. For 1 recipe,
    you can substitute 2 1/2–3 lb chicken parts for
    1 1/2 lb of skinless, boneless chicken breasts.)

Seasonings

salt (optional)
fresh ground pepper
dried basil
dried thyme
dried marjoram
dried oregano
bay leaf, 1
dried sage
Italian seasoning
dried minced onion (1/4 cup)

Staples

nonstick cooking spray
fresh or jar of chopped/minced garlic
canola oil
rice vinegar
granulated sugar
salad dressing (fat free or lite)

Miscellaneous

au jus gravy mix, 1 package

Breakfast foods:

_____

_____

_____

_____

_____

Lunch foods:

_____

_____

_____

_____

_____

Snack foods:

_____

_____

_____

_____

_____

Dinner Menus—Week 19 (No-Oven Menus)

Shrimp Salad • page 178
5 servings
whole-wheat roll*

Fajitas Barbecue Style • page 284
4 servings
Fruit Salad • page 159
8 servings

Chinese Chicken Salad • page 174
7 servings
Chocolate Mocha Mousse • page 308
8 servings

Grilled Salmon with Coconut-Cilantro Sauce • page 250
7 servings
eggplant slices* (cook on grill)

Tomato and Basil Pasta • page 203
4 servings
low-fat cottage cheese on lettuce leaf*

Week 19—Grocery List

Canned Vegetables/Sauces/Soups
(To lower sodium, choose no-added-salt or reduced-sodium products.)

bean sprouts (16 oz)
water chestnuts, sliced (8 oz)
coconut milk, lite (6 oz)—found in the
   Asian section

Pasta, Rice, & Beans
quick-cooking brown rice (1 1/2 cups)
angel hair pasta (6 oz)

Breads & Cereals
whole-wheat tortillas, 4 (8-inch) or 8 (6-inch)
whole-wheat rolls*

Fresh Produce
assorted fruit (4 cups)
avocado (1 medium)
minced fresh ginger (1 1/2 Tbsp)
fresh cilantro, chopped (1 1/4 cup)
salad greens, 10–12 oz (about 2 quarts)
shredded lettuce (1 cup)
tomatoes (5 medium)
Chinese Napa cabbage (1 small head)—
   1 1/2 lb
celery (1–2 stalks)
green onions (2 bunches)
eggplant*
6–10 lettuce leaves*
new potatoes (1 1/2 lb)—try Yukon gold

Dairy
cottage cheese, low fat*
yogurt, fat free, sugar free,
   fruit flavored (1 cup)
milk, fat free (3 cups)

Buy the amount for one meal or substitute a similar food.

Meat, Poultry, & Seafood
salad shrimp, cooked and cleaned (1 lb)
top sirloin steak, 1-inch thick (1 lb)
chicken breasts, skinless, boneless (1 lb)
salmon fillets (1 1/2 lb)

Seasonings
salt (optional)
fresh ground pepper
crushed red pepper
garlic powder
dried oregano
chili powder
ground ginger
dried basil

Staples
nonstick cooking spray
granulated sugar
rice vinegar (3/4 cup)
cider vinegar
lime juice (1/2 cup)
fresh or jar of chopped/minced garlic
canola oil
lite soy sauce
catsup
light brown sugar

Miscellaneous
dry-roasted peanuts, unsalted (1/2 cup)
ground fresh chili paste—1 tsp (optional)—
　　found in the Asian section
chocolate sugar-free instant pudding—
　　1 large box (2.1 oz)
instant coffee crystals (1 Tbsp)

Frozen
whipped topping, fat free (8 oz)

Breakfast foods:

_____

_____

_____

_____

_____

Lunch foods:

_____

_____

_____

_____

_____

Snack foods:

_____

_____

_____

_____

_____

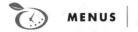

Dinner Menus—Week 20 (No-Oven Menus)

Chicken Picadillo • page 229
4 servings
whole-wheat tortilla*

Marinated Steak • page 285
6 servings
corn on the cob*
Cabbage Salad • page 167
6 servings

Oriental Rice and
Seafood Salad • page 175
5 servings
orange slices*

Grilled Chicken with
Fruit Salsa • page 240
4 servings
zucchini halves* (cook on grill)
whole-grain bread*

Clam Fettuccini • page 274
5 servings
tossed salad*

Week 20—Grocery List

Canned Vegetables/Sauces/Soups
(To lower sodium, choose no-added-salt or reduced-sodium products.)

salsa, thick and chunky (3/4 cup)
bean sprouts (16 oz)
water chestnuts, sliced (8 oz)

Canned Seafood
minced clams, 3 cans (6.5 oz each)

Pasta, Rice, & Beans
quick-cooking brown rice (1 1/2 cups)
fettuccini noodles, eggless (8 oz)

Breads & Cereals
whole-wheat tortillas*
whole-grain bread*

Fresh Produce
fresh fruit such as red papaya, nectarine,
    apricot, or peaches (2 cups cubed)
oranges*
onion (1 medium)
cabbage (1 small head)
celery (2 stalks)
avocado (1 medium)
green bell pepper (2 medium)
fresh cilantro, chopped (1/2 cup)
green onions (2 bunches)
corn on the cob*
zucchini*
salad fixings*

Buy the amount for one meal or substitute a similar food.

 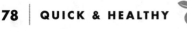

Meat, Poultry, & Seafood
chicken breasts, skinless, boneless (2 lb)
boneless steak, round, flank, or top sirloin
    (1 1/2 lb)
salad shrimp, cooked and cleaned (1 lb)

Seasonings
salt (optional)
fresh ground pepper
ground cumin
dried parsley
dried oregano
garlic powder
chili powder
ground mustard
dried thyme
toasted sesame seeds (3 tablespoons)

Staples
nonstick cooking spray
fresh or jar of chopped/minced garlic
Worcestershire sauce
rice vinegar (1/2 cup)
lite soy sauce
granulated sugar
lime juice
lemon juice
salad dressing (fat free or lite)

Breakfast foods:

_____

_____

_____

_____

_____

Lunch foods:

_____

_____

_____

_____

_____

Snack foods:

_____

_____

_____

_____

_____

More Menus

On the next pages are recipes from this book grouped by what food can be added to make a balanced meal. Refer to the food groups below for more choices

Food Groups

Starch
Breads, crackers, bagels, bulgur, couscous, pasta, polenta, quinoa, rice, tortillas, dried beans, peas, lentils

Starchy vegetables
Corn, hominy, parsnips, peas, potatoes, succotash, winter squash, yams

Nonstarchy vegetables
Salad greens, asparagus, artichokes, broccoli, Brussels sprouts, cabbage, carrots, cauliflower, celery, cucumbers, eggplant, green and wax beans, cooked greens, jicama, mushrooms, onions, pea pods, peppers, radishes, sauerkraut, spinach, summer squash, tomatoes, water chestnuts, zucchini

Protein
Lean meat, poultry, and seafood; reduced fat and low-fat cheeses, eggs, and egg substitutes

For the section on menus that includes 20 weeks of balanced dinner menus (with side dishes included) and the grocery list, go to page 38. Also visit www.QuickandHealthy.net for more dinner menus.

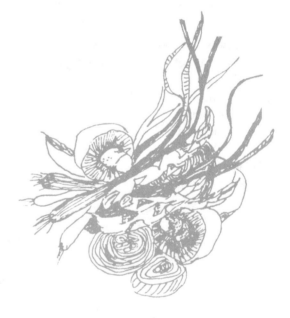

Serve Alone or Add a Salad

The following recipes contain starch, nonstarchy vegetable, and protein. Serve alone or complete the meal with a nonstarchy vegetable, such as a salad or raw vegetable slices.

Poultry
Chicken and Artichokes Dijon
Chicken and Rice Casserole
Mediterranean Chicken
Mexican-Style Chicken and Rice
Chicken Fajitas

Beef or Pork
Fajitas Barbecue Style
Beef or Pork Fajitas
Pork and Rice Casserole

Seafood
Mediterranean Seafood

Ground Meat
Creamy Cabbage Stir-Fry
John Torrey
Tortilla Pie
Asparagus-Topped Meatloaf

Soups
Thai Chicken Soup
Chicken Curry Soup
Tortilla Soup
Taco Soup
Sausage and Bean Soup
Chili Con Carne

Add a Salad or Raw Vegetable Sticks

The following recipes contain starch and protein. Serve with a nonstarchy vegetable such as celery and carrot sticks or a tossed salad.

Meatless
Quick Lasagna

Poultry
Chicken Tortilla Casserole
Baked Chimichangas
Chicken Enchiladas
Green Chile Chicken Enchilada Casserole
Chicken and Biscuits
Chicken in a Pocket
Turkey French Dips

Seafood
Clam Fettuccini
Grilled Salmon with Coconut-
   Cilantro Sauce
Boboli Pizza Shrimp Style
New England Fish Chowder

Ground Meat
Spaghetti and Meatballs
Meatball Sandwich
Biscuits and Gravy
Moore
Quick Meat and Bean Supper
Quick Meat Lasagna
Crusty Calzone
Sloppy Joes

Serve Alone or Add a Whole-Grain Roll

The following recipes contain starch, nonstarchy vegetable, and protein. Serve alone or complete the meal with a whole-grain roll or another whole-grain product.

Chinese Chicken Salad
Oriental Rice and Seafood Salad
Sausage and Sauerkraut

Add a Whole-Grain Roll

The following recipes contain protein and fruit or nonstarchy vegetable. Serve with a whole-grain roll or another whole-grain product.

Curry Tuna Salad
Cinnamon Chicken Salad
Chicken and Fruit Salad
Chicken and Spinach Salad
Shrimp Salad
Italian Cioppino
Chilled Tomato-Shrimp Soup
Barbecued Smoked Sausage and
   Cabbage Casserole
Italian Zucchini Frittata
Spanish Zucchini Frittata

Add a Starch (Starchy Vegetable, Noodles, or Brown Rice)

The following recipes contain fruit or nonstarchy vegetables and protein. Serve with a starch, such as noodles, brown rice, or a starchy vegetable (corn, peas, or potatoes). Another choice is to add a whole-grain roll or another whole-grain product.

Poultry
Spicy Chicken and Grapes
Sweet and Sour Chicken
Chicken and Broccoli Casserole
Chicken Breasts Florentine
Chicken Cacciatore
Rolled Chicken and Asparagus
Teriyaki Chicken Stir-Fry
Chicken and Pea Pod Stir-Fry
Chicken and Vegetables in Gravy
Mandarin Orange Chicken
Chicken Picadillo

Beef and Pork
Pork or Beef Stir-Fry
Chinese Pepper Steak
Pork Chop Suey
Orange Pork Chops

Seafood
Spanish Baked Fish
Mandarin Orange Seafood
Spicy Seafood with Grapes

Add a Nonstarchy Vegetable and a Starch

The following recipes contain mostly protein. To balance the meal, add a nonstarchy vegetable, either cooked or raw. Also add a starch, such as noodles, brown rice, whole-grain roll, or a starchy vegetable, such as corn, peas, or potatoes.

Poultry
Polynesian Chicken
Oven-Fried Chicken
Chicken in Salsa
Yogurt Cumin Chicken
Chicken Breasts in Mushroom Sauce
Chicken Breasts Supreme
Chicken Nuggets
Crispy Potato Chicken
French Glazed Chicken
Hickory-Smoked Barbecued Chicken
Grilled Chicken with Coconut-
   Cilantro Sauce
Grilled Chicken with Corn Salsa
Grilled Chicken with Fruit Salsa
Chicken Lettuce Wraps

Ground Meat
Pizza Meat Loaf
Meat Patties
Meat Loaf
Swedish Meatballs
Turkey Lettuce Wraps
Beef Lettuce Wraps
Crustless Quiche

Seafood
Polynesian Fish
Fillets of Sole Thermidor
Lemon Fish
Oven-Fried Fish
Poached Fish
Salmon Cakes
Sweet Mustard Fish
Tarragon Fish
Yogurt Cumin Fish
French Glazed Fish
Hickory-Smoked Barbecued Fish
Grilled Fish with Fruit Salsa
Grilled Salmon with Corn Salsa
Shrimp Lettuce Wraps
Fish in Salsa

Beef and Pork
Marinated Steak
Oven-Fried Pork Loin

Add a Protein

The following recipes contain nonstarchy vegetables and starch. To add additional protein, include a serving of a low-fat or reduced-fat cheese, fat-free yogurt, or fat-free milk. You may also want to add a raw vegetable or a roll.

Minestrone Soup
Oriental Noodle Soup
Three-Bean Soup
Italian Broccoli and Pasta
Tomato and Basil Pasta
Piled-High Vegetable Pizza

Recipes Listed by Carbohydrate

Following is a table, listing recipes that are grouped by grams of carbohydrate. This can be especially helpful for people with diabetes when planning meals around a specific number of grams of carbohydrate. It is also helpful for people in weight loss programs who need calories, grams of fat, and dietary fiber for their calculations.

You can adjust your serving size, which will increase or decrease the grams of carbohydrate per serving, to meet your individual needs.

This listing includes calories, fat, carbohydrate, carb servings, and fiber.

Some recipes are listed twice if the nutrient analysis is provided for both artificial sweetener and regular sugar.

Carb servings listed have been adjusted for fiber. In some recipes this resulted in no change. If the fiber is more than 5 grams, half of the grams of fiber are subtracted from the total grams of carbohydrate when figuring exchanges and carb servings.

Below is the number of recipes listed by grams of carbohydrate in the table that follows:

52 recipes	0–5 grams of carbohydrate
43 recipes	6–10 grams of carbohydrate
66 recipes	11–20 grams of carbohydrate
35 recipes	21–25 grams of carbohydrate
36 recipes	26–35 grams of carbohydrate
5 recipes	36–40 grams of carbohydrate

Recipes Listed by Grams of Carbohydrate

One portion of the following recipes has 0-5 grams of carbohydrate and is counted as 0 Carb Servings.

	One Serving	Calories	Total Fat grams	Carbo-hydrate grams	Dietary Fiber grams	Carb Servings
APPETIZERS						
Beef Lettuce Wraps – 1 wrap	1 wrap	59	3	1	0	0
Chinese Barbecued Pork	2 slices(1oz pork)	47	2	2	0	0
Cottage Cheese Dip and Topping	2 Tbsps	15	0	1	0	0
Creamy Seafood Dip	2 Tbsps	22	0	1	0	0
Hot Artichoke and Spinach Dip	1/4 cup	70	4	4	2	0
Shrimp Lettuce Wraps – 1 wrap	1 wrap	43	0	1	0	0
Shrimp Lettuce Wraps – 1 wrap*	1 wrap	40	0	1	0	0
Smoked Salmon Spread	2 Tbsps	38	1	1	0	0
Spinach Dip	1/4 cup	42	2	5	1	0
Turkey Lettuce Wraps – 1 wrap	1 wrap	62	3	2	1	0
BEVERAGES						
Cran-Raspberry Cooler	1 cup	15	0	4	0	0
GRAVIES, SAUCES, & MARINADES						
Cornstarch Gravy	2 Tbsps	6	0	1	0	0
Flour Gravy	2 Tbsps	9	0	2	0	0
Fresh Cucumber Sauce for Seafood	1/4 cup	37	3	3	0	0
Fruit Sauce*	1/4 cup	19	0	4	3	0
Seafood Marinade – Lemon Basil Marinade	1 Tbsp	32	3	1	0	0
Seafood Marinade – Soy Marinade	1/2 Tbsp	24	2	0	0	0
Spanish Yogurt Sauce	1/4 cup	27	0	4	0	0
Thick and Chunky Salsa	1/4 cup	14	0	3	1	0
VEGETABLES						
Baked Portobello Mushrooms	1 mushroom	32	1	4	1	0
Basil Tomatoes	1/2 cup	18	0	4	1	0
Gourmet Cucumbers	1/2 cup	23	0	5	0	0
Gourmet Cucumbers*	1/2 cup	14	0	3	0	0
Italian Tomatoes	1/2 cup	19	0	5	1	0
Marinated Vegetables	1/2 cup	19	1	3	1	0
Seasoned Green Beans*	1/3 cup	26	0	5	2	0

*Indicates artificial sweetener used. This recipe is listed again without using artificial sweetener.

	One Serving	Calories	Total Fat grams	Carbo-hydrate grams	Dietary Fiber grams	Carb Servings
SALADS						
Greek Salad	1 cup	33	0	5	1	0
POULTRY						
Chicken in Salsa	1/4th	138	1	3	0	0
Chicken Lettuce Wraps – 1 wrap	1 wrap	44	1	1	0	0
Chicken Lettuce Wraps – 3 wraps	3 wraps	131	2	2	1	0
Cooked and Cubed Chicken	1/2 cup	108	1	0	0	0
Hickory-Smoked Barbecued Chicken	1/4th	127	1	0	0	0
Oven-Fried Chicken	1/6th	137	1	3	0	0
Polynesian Chicken*	1/4th	134	2	1	0	0
Yogurt Cumin Chicken	1/4th	143	2	5	0	0
SEAFOOD						
Fillets of Sole Thermidor	1/8th	146	3	3	0	0
Fish in Salsa	1/4th	128	2	3	0	0
Hickory-Smoked Barbecued Fish	1/4th	164	7	0	0	0
Lemon Fish	1/4th	116	2	1	0	0
Oven-Fried Fish	1/4th	134	2	5	0	0
Poached Fish	1/4th	120	2	1	0	0
Polynesian Fish*	1/4th	171	7	1	0	0
Shrimp Lettuce Wraps – 3 wraps	3 wraps	129	1	4	1	0
Shrimp Lettuce Wraps – 3 wraps*	3 wraps	121	1	2	1	0
Sweet Mustard Fish*	1/4th	131	2	2	0	0
Tarragon Fish	1/4th	146	3	2	0	0
Yogurt Cumin Fish	1/4th	132	2	5	0	0
BEEF AND PORK						
Marinated Steak	1/6th	183	9	1	0	0
Oven-Fried Pork Loin	1/4th	167	5	5	0	0
GROUND MEAT AND SAUSAGE						
Beef Lettuce Wraps – 3 wraps	3 wraps	177	8	4	1	0
Pizza Meat Loaf	1/4th	172	8	2	1	0
DESSERTS						
Cream Cheese Topping	2 Tbsps	21	0	3	0	0

*Indicates artificial sweetener used. This recipe is listed again without using artificial sweetener.

 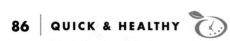

One portion of the following recipes has 6–10 grams of carbohydrate and is counted as 1/2 Carb Serving.

	One Serving	Calories	Total Fat grams	Carbo- hydrate grams	Dietary Fiber grams	Carb Servings
GRAVIES & SAUCES						
Fruit Sauce	1/4 cup	32	0	8	3	1/2
SOUPS & STEWS						
Vegetable Soup	1 1/4 cups	36	0	6	2	1/2
VEGETABLES						
Roasted Eggplant Medley	1/2 cup	30	0	7	3	1/2
Salsa Vegetables	1/2 cup	28	0	6	1	1/2
Seasoned Green Beans	1/3 cup	28	0	6	2	1/2
Zucchini, Tomato, and Onion	1/2 cup	29	0	7	2	1/2
SALADS						
Apple Salad Mold	1/2 cup	39	0	8	1	1/2
Broccoli Salad	1 cup	68	4	6	3	1/2
Cabbage Salad	1 cup	54	2	9	3	1/2
Cabbage Salad*	1 cup	45	2	7	3	1/2
Cinnamon Chicken Salad	1 cup	169	5	10	1	1/2
Curry Tuna Salad	3/4 cup	165	6	7	1	1/2
Italian Garden Salad	3/4 cup	28	0	6	1	1/2
Italian Zucchini Frittata	1/4th	65	1	6	1	1/2
Mexican Garden Salad	3/4 cup	97	7	10	4	1/2
Seafood Salad	1/2 cup	85	3	7	0	1/2
Shrimp Coleslaw	1 cup	86	1	10	2	1/2
Shrimp Coleslaw*	1 cup	80	1	8	2	1/2
Shrimp Salad*	2 1/2 cups	228	12	9	5	1/2
Spanish Zucchini Frittata	1/4th	59	0	7	2	1/2
Three-Bean Salad*	1/2 cup	62	1	13	6	1/2**
Vegetable Bean Salad*	1/2 cup	44	0	9	4	1/2
POULTRY						
Chicken and Broccoli Casserole	1/5th	168	3	10	4	1/2
Chicken Breasts Florentine	1/6th	164	2	6	2	1/2
Chicken Breasts in Mushroom Sauce	1/4th	170	2	8	1	1/2
Chicken Breasts Supreme	1/8th	162	1	6	0	1/2
Chicken Nuggets	1/4th	164	1	9	0	1/2
Chicken Picadillo	1/4th	165	2	9	1	1/2

*Indicates artificial sweetener used. This recipe is listed again without using artificial sweetener.

**Carb servings listed have been adjusted for fiber. In some recipes this resulted in no change. If the fiber is more than 5 grams, half of the grams of fiber are subtracted from the total grams of carbohydrate when figuring exchanges and carb servings.

	One Serving	Calories	Total Fat grams	Carbo-hydrate grams	Dietary Fiber grams	Carb Servings
Crispy Potato Chicken	1/4th	167	3	6	1	1/2
French Glazed Chicken	1/4th	155	1	9	0	1/2
Grilled Chicken with Corn Salsa	1/2 cup salsa, 1/8 chicken	152	2	6	1	1/2
Rolled Chicken and Asparagus	1/4th	151	2	6	3	1/2
Teriyaki Chicken Stir-Fry	1 1/2 cups	210	6	10	3	1/2
SEAFOOD						
French Glazed Fish	1/4th	145	2	9	0	1/2
Grilled Salmon with Corn Salsa	1/2 cup salsa, 1/8 fish	189	7	6	1	1/2
Salmon Cakes	1 cake	181	9	6	0	1/2
Spanish Baked Fish	1/4th	137	2	6	1	1/2
BEEF AND PORK						
Beef or Pork Stir-Fry	1/4th	213	9	8	3	1/2
GROUND MEAT AND SAUSAGE						
Baked Meatballs	4 meatballs	146	6	6	1	1/2
Crustless Quiche with Ground Meat	1/6th	120	3	6	0	1/2
Meat Patties	1 patty	222	9	9	1	1/2
Turkey Lettuce Wraps – 3 wraps	3 wraps	192	8	7	2	1/2
DESSERTS						
Lemon Parfait	3/4 cup	55	0	10	0	1/2

One portion of the following recipes has 11–20 grams of carbohydrates and is counted as 1 Carb Serving.

BEVERAGES						
Banana Milk Shake*	1 cup	99	0	20	1	1
Buttermilk Fruit Shake	1 cup	100	1	18	2	1
Buttermilk Fruit Shake*	1 cup	85	1	14	2	1
Fruit Milk Shake	1 cup	96	0	19	2	1
Fruit Milk Shake*	1 cup	80	0	14	2	1
BREADS						
Cottage Cheese Pancakes*	2 pancakes	119	1	17	3	1
Dumplings	1 dumpling	85	0	17	2	1
Italian Focaccia Bread	1 slice	104	1	20	1	1
Oat Bran Muffins	1 muffin	121	4	20	3	1

*Indicates artificial sweetener used. This recipe is listed again without using artificial sweetener.

	One Serving	Calories	Total Fat grams	Carbo-hydrate grams	Dietary Fiber grams	Carb Servings
SOUPS & STEWS						
Chilled Tomato-Shrimp Soup	1 1/2 cups	129	1	11	1	1
Gazpacho	1 1/2 cups	91	3	16	3	1
Minestrone Soup	1 cup	110	1	20	5	1
Oriental Noodle Soup	1 cup	79	1	14	1	1
SALADS						
Chicken and Fruit Salad	1 1/2 cups	173	3	19	3	1
Chicken and Spinach Salad	2 3/4 cups	190	7	16	4	1
Fruit Salad	1/2 cup	60	0	14	1	1
Grapefruit & Avocado Salad	2 cups	134	8	16	5	1
Grapefruit & Avocado Salad*	2 cups	128	8	14	5	1
Herb Potato Salad	1 cup	74	1	14	2	1
Lime Cottage Salad	3/4 cup	121	1	16	0	1
Macaroni Salad*	3/4 cup	134	5	19	2	1
Romaine & Mandarin Orange Salad	2 cups	140	8	17	4	1
Romaine & Mandarin Orange Salad*	2 cups	125	8	13	4	1
Shrimp Salad	2 1/2 cups	247	12	14	5	1
Three-Bean Salad	1/2 cup	70	1	15	6	1**
Vegetable Bean Salad	1/2 cup	52	0	11	4	1
POTATOES, RICE, & BEANS						
Cheese-Stuffed Potatoes—1% cot chse	1 potato half	71	0	12	2	1
Sweet Potato Fries	1/4th	116	4	20	3	1
SANDWICHES & PIZZA						
Individual Pizza	1 pizza	159	3	16	3	1
Tomato and Ricotta Sandwich	1 sandwich	138	3	20	4	1
POULTRY						
Chicken and Pea Pod Stir-Fry	1/4th	188	2	14	4	1
Chicken and Vegetables in Gravy	1/6th	192	2	11	4	1
Chicken Cacciatore	1/6th	197	2	15	4	1
Grilled Chicken with Coconut-Cilantro Sauce*	1/5th	216	4	19	1	1
Grilled Chicken with Fruit Salsa	1 cup salsa, 1/4 chicken	230	8	13	5	1
Mandarin Orange Chicken	1 cup	194	2	16	3	1
Polynesian Chicken	1/4th	186	2	14	0	1
Spicy Chicken and Grapes	1 cup	172	1	17	2	1

*Indicates artificial sweetener used. This recipe is listed again without using artificial sweetener.

**Carb servings listed have been adjusted for fiber. In some recipes this resulted in no change. If the fiber is more than 5 grams, half of the grams of fiber are subtracted from the total grams of carbohydrate when figuring exchanges and carb servings.

	One Serving	Calories	Total Fat grams	Carbo-hydrate grams	Dietary Fiber grams	Carb Servings
Spicy Chicken and Grapes*	1 cup	162	1	15	2	1
Sweet and Sour Chicken*	1 cup	152	1	12	2	1
SEAFOOD						
Grilled Salmon with Coconut-Cilantro Sauce*	1/7th	229	8	17	3	1
Grilled Salmon with Coconut-Cilantro Sauce	1/7th	237	8	19	3	1
Grilled Salmon with Fruit Salsa	1 cup salsa, 1/8 fish	264	14	12	5	1
Mandarin Orange Seafood	1 cup	171	1	19	3	1
Oven-Fried Oysters	1/4th	110	2	13	0	1
Polynesian Fish	1/4th	223	7	14	0	1
Sweet Mustard Fish	1/4th	162	2	11	0	1
BEEF AND PORK						
Chinese Pepper Steak	1 1/4 cup	254	9	16	3	1
Chinese Pepper Steak*	1 1/4 cup	252	9	16	3	1
Orange Pork Chops	1/4th	223	8	13	3	1
Pork Chop Suey	1 1/4 cups	219	5	16	2	1
Sausage and Sauerkraut	about 1 1/2 cups	230	8	22	6	1**
GROUND MEAT & SAUSAGE						
Asparagus-Topped Meatloaf	1/4th	286	10	19	4	1
Barbecued-Smoked Sausage & Cabbage Casserole	about 1 cup	203	8	17	3	1
Meat Loaf	1/6th	244	9	16	2	1
Swedish Meatballs	5 meatballs, 1/4 cup sauce	214	8	13	2	1
DESSERTS						
Apple Cake*	1/16th	110	4	17	2	1
Apple Crisp	1/8th	88	1	19	2	1
Apple Crisp*	1/8th	68	1	14	2	1
Chocolate Mocha Mousse	3/4 cup	104	0	20	1	1
Coffee Mousse	3/4 cup	98	0	19	0	1
Fruit Slush	1 cup	91	0	17	4	1
Fruit Slush*	1 cup	74	0	13	4	1
Mandarin Orange Cake*	1/9th	112	3	18	1	1
Peppermint Mousse	3/4 cup	102	0	19	0	1
White Chocolate Mousse with Berries	3/4 cup	78	0	16	2	1

*Indicates artificial sweetener used. This recipe is listed again without using artificial sweetener.

**Carb servings listed have been adjusted for fiber. In some recipes this resulted in no change. If the fiber is more than 5 grams, half of the grams of fiber are subtracted from the total grams of carbohydrate when figuring exchanges and carb servings.

One portion of the following recipes has 21–25 grams of carbohydrate and is counted as 1 1/2 Carb Servings.

	One Serving	Calories	Total Fat grams	Carbo- hydrate grams	Dietary Fiber grams	Carb Servings
BEVERAGES						
Banana Milk Shake	1 cup	115	0	24	1	1 1/2
Orange Julius	3/4 cup	113	0	22	0	1 1/2
BREADS						
Applesauce Oatmeal Coffee Cake	1 piece	164	5	25	2	1 1/2
Blueberry Coffee Cake	1 piece	156	5	24	2	1 1/2
Cottage Cheese Pancakes	2 pancakes	135	1	22	3	1 1/2
Refrigerator Bran Muffins	1 muffin	141	5	25	4	1 1/2
SOUPS & STEWS						
Chicken Curry Soup	2 cups	248	2	24	2	1 1/2
Chili Con Carne	1 cup	242	6	27	11	1 1/2**
Italian Cioppino	1 1/2 cups	207	2	22	4	1 1/2
New England Fish Chowder	1 1/2 cups	220	2	22	2	1 1/2
Three-Bean Soup	1 cup	124	1	25	8	1 1/2**
SALADS						
Chinese Chicken Salad	2 cups	213	6	24	3	1 1/2
Chinese Chicken Salad*	2 cups	209	6	23	3	1 1/2
Macaroni Salad	3/4 cup	141	5	21	2	1 1/2
Pear Salad with Raspberry Dressing	2 cups	158	7	23	5	1 1/2
POTATOES, RICE, & BEANS						
Low-Fat French Fries	1/4th	129	4	22	3	1 1/2
Roasted Root Vegetables	1 cup	131	4	23	4	1 1/2
Scalloped Potatoes	2/3 cup	107	0	22	3	1 1/2
MEATLESS ENTREES						
Italian Broccoli and Pasta	1/4th	109	1	22	3	1 1/2
POULTRY						
Chicken and Rice Casserole	1/4th	247	2	25	4	1 1/2
Grilled Chicken with Coconut-Cilantro Sauce	1/5th	226	4	23	1	1 1/2
Mediterranean Chicken	1 1/2 cups	213	2	25	3	1 1/2
Mexican-Style Chicken and Rice	1/5th	241	4	25	3	1 1/2
Sweet and Sour Chicken	1 cup	193	1	23	2	1 1/2

*Indicates artificial sweetener used. This recipe is listed again without using artificial sweetener.

**Carb servings listed have been adjusted for fiber. In some recipes this resulted in no change. If the fiber is more than 5 grams, half of the grams of fiber are subtracted from the total grams of carbohydrate when figuring exchanges and carb servings.

SEAFOOD	One Serving	Calories	Total Fat grams	Carbo- hydrate grams	Dietary Fiber grams	Carb Servings
Spicy Seafood with Grapes*	1 1/4 cups	179	1	21	2	1 1/2
Spicy Seafood with Grapes	1 1/4 cups	192	1	24	2	1 1/2
GROUND MEAT AND SAUSAGE						
Quick Meat and Bean Supper	1 cup	293	8	26	6	1 1/2**
DESSERTS						
Apple Cake	1/16th	142	4	25	2	1 1/2
Butterfly Cup Cakes	1 filled cupcake	140	4	23	1	1 1/2
Fruit Pizza Cookies	1 cookie	155	5	25	1	1 1/2
Fruit Pizza for a Crowd	1/18th	155	5	25	1	1 1/2
Grasshopper Mousse	3/4 cup	115	0	22	0	1 1/2
Mandarin Orange Cake	1/9th	134	3	24	1	1 1/2
Pineapple Cake*		96	0	21	1	1 1/2
Strawberries Romanoff	1 cup	106	1	23	3	1 1/2

One portion of the following recipes has 26–35 grams of carbohydrates and is counted as 2 Carb Servings.

SOUPS & STEWS						
Quick & Healthy Tortilla Soup	2 cups	241	3	37	7	2**
Sausage and Bean Soup	1 1/2 cups	261	6	38	12	2**
Taco Soup	1 1/2 cups	285	6	40	10	2**
Thai Chicken Soup	1 3/4 cups	233	2	28	3	2
POTATOES, RICE, & BEANS						
Herb and Vegetable Rice Blend	3/4 cup	142	1	27	2	2
Herb Rice Blend	1/2 cup	136	1	26	2	2
Ranch Beans	1/2 cup	160	0	31	9	2**
SANDWICHES & PIZZA						
Boboli Pizza Shrimp Style	2 slices	259	6	28	1	2
Crusty Calzone – Ground Meat	1 slice	230	6	29	3	2
Crusty Calzone – Turkey Sausage	1 slice	237	7	30	3	2
Piled-High Vegetable Pizza	2 slices	238	6	34	5	2
Turkey French Dips	1 sandwich	273	5	31	4	2
SALADS						
Oriental Rice and Seafood Salad*	1 1/2 cups	225	2	28	3	2
Oriental Rice and Seafood Salad	1 1/2 cups	235	2	30	3	2

*Indicates artificial sweetener used. This recipe is listed again without using artificial sweetener.

**Carb servings listed have been adjusted for fiber. In some recipes this resulted in no change. If the fiber is more than 5 grams, half of the grams of fiber are subtracted from the total grams of carbohydrate when figuring exchanges and carb servings.

 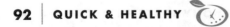

	One Serving	Calories	Total Fat grams	Carbo-hydrate grams	Dietary Fiber grams	Carb Servings
MEATLESS ENTREES						
Quick Lasagna	1/12th	218	5	28	2	2
Vegetables Primavera	1/5th	169	3	29	5	2
POULTRY						
Baked Chimichangas	1/4th	260	5	27	2	2
Chicken and Artichokes Dijon	1/4th	316	7	28	5	2
Chicken and Artichokes Dijon*	1/4th	308	7	26	5	2
Chicken and Biscuits	2 biscuits, 1/5th casserole	261	3	31	3	2
Chicken Enchiladas	1/8th	237	6	26	3	2
Chicken Fajitas	1/4th	278	3	30	3	2
Chicken in a Pocket	1 roll	249	4	26	2	2
Chicken Tortilla Casserole	1/10th	274	6	30	3	2
Green Chile Chicken Enchilada Casserole	1/8th	281	8	27	2	2
SEAFOOD						
Mediterranean Seafood	1 3/4 cups	249	2	32	4	2
BEEF AND PORK						
Beef or Pork Fajitas	1/4th	332	10	30	3	2
Fajitas Barbecue Style	1/4th	326	10	28	3	2
Pork and Rice Casserole	1 cup	297	7	30	3	2
GROUND MEAT & SAUSAGE						
Biscuits and Gravy	2 biscuits, 2/3 cup gravy	292	11	28	1	2
John Torrey	about 1 cup	290	8	31	3	2
Quick Meat Lasagna	1/12th	265	7	29	2	2
Spaghetti and Meatballs	4 meatballs, 1/2 cup noodles with sauce	277	9	28	4	2
Tortilla Pie	1/10th	288	9	31	3	2
DESSERTS						
Cherry Cream Cheese Dessert	3/4 cup	142	2	26	1	2
Pineapple Cake	1/16th	121	0	28	1	2

*Indicates artificial sweetener used. This recipe is listed again without using artificial sweetener.

One portion of the following recipes has 36–40 grams of carbohydrates and is counted as 2 1/2 Carb Servings.

SANDWICHES & PIZZA	One Serving	Calories	Total Fat grams	Carbo-hydrate grams	Dietary Fiber grams	Carb Servings
Meatball Sandwich	1 sandwich	331	10	40	6	2 1/2**
Sloppy Joes	1 sandwich	336	10	40	5	2 1/2
MEATLESS ENTREES						
Tomato and Basil Pasta	1 1/2 cups	193	1	39	4	2 1/2
SEAFOOD						
Clam Fettuccini	1 cup	225	1	37	2	2 1/2
GROUND MEAT AND SAUSAGE						
Creamy Cabbage Stir-Fry	2 cups	345	9	39	5	2 1/2

One portion of the following recipes has 41–50 grams of carbohydrates and is counted as 3 Carb Servings.

GROUND MEAT AND SAUSAGE	One Serving	Calories	Total Fat grams	Carbo-hydrate grams	Dietary Fiber grams	Carb Servings
Moore	1 1/4 cups	374	10	41	2	3

**Carb servings listed have been adjusted for fiber. In some recipes this resulted in no change. If the fiber is more than 5 grams, half of the grams of fiber are subtracted from the total grams of carbohydrate when figuring exchanges and carb servings.

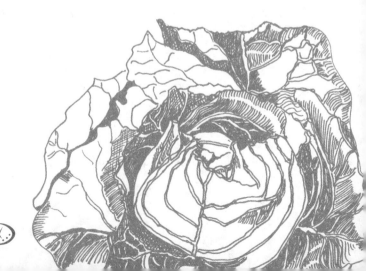

Measurements and Metric Conversions

Standard Measures

3 teaspoons	=	1 tablespoon
4 tablespoons	=	1/4 cup
8 tablespoons	=	1/2 cup
16 tablespoons	=	1 cup
1 cup	=	8 ounces, fluid
2 cups	=	1 pint
4 cups	=	1 quart
4 quarts	=	1 gallon
16 ounces	=	1 pound

Weights

U.S.		Metric
1 oz	=	28 g
2 oz	=	57 g
4 oz (1/4 lb)	=	114 g
6 oz	=	170 g
8 oz (1/2 lb)	=	227 g
12 oz (3/4 lb)	=	340 g
1 lb (16 oz)	=	454 g

Length

U.S.		Metric
1 inch	=	2.54 cm
8 inches	=	20 cm
9 inches	=	23 cm
13 inches	=	33 cm

Figures based on

1 oz	=	28.35 g
1 lb	=	453.59 g
1 Tbsp	=	14.8 ml
1 cup	=	237 ml

Volume

U.S.		Metric
1/4 tsp	=	1 ml
1/2 tsp	=	2 ml
1 tsp	=	5 ml
2 tsp	=	10 ml
1 Tbsp	=	15 ml
1/4 cup (4 Tbsp)	=	60 ml
1/3 cup	=	80 ml
1/2 cup (8 Tbsp)	=	120 ml
2/3 cup	=	160 ml
3/4 cup	=	180 ml
1 cup (16 Tbsp)	=	240 ml
2 cups	=	480 ml
4 cups (1 quart)	=	950 ml

Temperatures

Fahrenheit		Celsius
325	=	165
350	=	175
375	=	190
400	=	205
425	=	220
450	=	230

Abbreviations

oz	=	ounce
lb	=	pound
tsp	=	teaspoon
Tbsp	=	tablespoon
qt	=	quart
g	=	grams
ml	=	milliliter
cm	=	centimeter
l	=	liter

Beverages

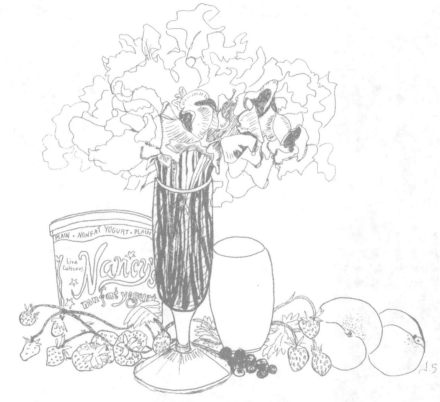

In this section, you'll find refreshing drinks for hot summer days and an assortment of blended drinks that are great for a snack or an addition to a healthy breakfast.

This popular breakfast drink can also be served as a delicious after-school snack.

Makes 4 1/2 cups
6 servings

Each Serving
3/4 cup

Carb Servings
1 1/2

Exchanges
1 fruit
1/2 fat-free milk

Nutrient Analysis
calories 113
total fat 0g
saturated fat 0g
cholesterol 3mg
sodium 74mg
total carbohydrate 22g
dietary fiber 0g
sugars 21g
protein 6g

Orange Julius

2 1/2 cups fat-free milk
8 ounces fat-free plain yogurt
6 ounces frozen orange juice concentrate
1 teaspoon vanilla extract

Process all ingredients in a blender until smooth.

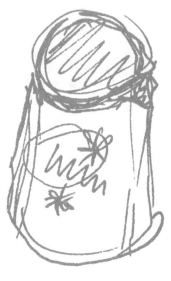

Fruit Milk Shake

1/2 cup fat-free milk or fat-free plain yogurt
1/2 cup sliced fruit (peaches, strawberries, etc.)
2 ice cubes
1/2 teaspoon vanilla extract
sweetener to taste: 1–2 teaspoons sugar or the equivalent
   in artificial sweetener

Process the first four ingredients in a blender until
smooth. Sweeten to taste.

NOTE: For a more creamy texture, use yogurt instead of
        milk. Frozen fruit can be substituted for fresh and
        the ice cubes can be eliminated.

*Take advantage of
seasonal fresh fruit
when making this recipe.*

Makes 1 serving

Each Serving

Carb Servings
1

Exchanges
1 fruit—1/2 with artificial
   sweetener
1/2 fat-free milk

Nutrient Analysis
calories 96—with artificial
   sweetener 80
total fat 0g
saturated fat 0g
cholesterol 2mg
sodium 51mg
total carbohydrate 19g—
   with artificial sweetener
   14g
dietary fiber 2g
sugars 18g—with artificial
   sweetener 14g
protein 5g

Burgundy wine with Fresca combine to give a good flavor and a berry pink color. If you prefer less sweetness, use half Fresca and half tonic water. Garnish with orange or lemon slice.

Makes 1 serving

Each Serving

Carb Servings
0

Exchanges
1 alcohol equivalent

Nutrient Analysis
calories 80
total fat 0g
saturated fat 0g
cholesterol 0mg
sodium 41mg
total carbohydrate 1g
dietary fiber 0g
sugars 0g
protein 0g

Wine Cooler

1 cup sugar-free soda pop (Fresca, lemon lime, ginger ale, tonic water, Sprite, Club Soda, seltzer water, etc.)
1/2 cup wine (white, red, or blush)
ice cubes

Fill a tall glass with ice cubes. Add soda pop and wine. Stir to mix.

Banana Milk Shake

1/2 small banana
1/2 cup fat-free milk
1/4 teaspoon almond extract
2 ice cubes (optional)
sweetener to taste: 1 teaspoon sugar or the equivalent in
   artificial sweetener

Process the first four ingredients in a blender until
smooth. Sweeten to taste.

NOTE: Use frozen bananas to give an ice cream–like
      texture. Start with fresh bananas and freeze them
      in the peel. The frozen peel will turn black but
      the inside will remain a creamy white. Let them
      set out at room temperature about 10 minutes for
      easier peeling.

*Take advantage of
bananas on sale and freeze
to have several on hand.*

Makes 1 serving

Each Serving

Carb Servings
1 1/2—with artificial
   sweetener 1

Exchanges
1 fruit
1/2 fat-free milk

Nutrient Analysis
calories 115—with
   artificial sweetener 99
total fat 0g
saturated fat 0g
cholesterol 2mg
sodium 52mg
total carbohydrate 24g—
   with artificial sweetener
   20g
dietary fiber 1g
sugars 18g—with artificial
   sweetener 13g
protein 5g

This is a refreshing drink that is also a pretty pink color. Be sure to look for the light version of the cranberry juice, as it has two-thirds less calories and sugar than the regular version.

Makes 1 serving

Each Serving

Carb Servings
0

Exchanges
free

Nutrient Analysis
calories 15
total fat 0g
saturated fat 0g
cholesterol 0mg
sodium 23mg
total carbohydrate 4g
dietary fiber 0g
sugars 4g
protein 0g

Cran-Raspberry Cooler

1/2 cup diet Squirt
1/2 cup light cran-raspberry juice drink
ice cubes

Fill a tall glass with ice. Add Squirt and juice. Enjoy!

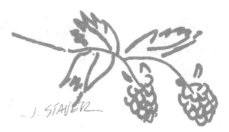

J. STAVER

Juice Cooler

1 cup sugar-free soda pop (lemon lime, Sprite, tonic
   water, Fresca, etc.)
1/2 cup fruit juice, unsweetened
ice cubes

Fill a tall glass with ice cubes. Add soda pop and juice.
Stir to mix.

Try this recipe with orange juice and lemon soda or use other juices for variety. Garnish with lemon or lime slice.

Makes 1 serving

Each Serving

Carb Servings
1

Exchanges
1 fruit

Nutrient Analysis
calories 56
total fat 0g
saturated fat 0g
cholesterol 0mg
sodium 36mg
total carbohydrate 13g
dietary fiber 0g
sugars 10g
protein 1g

Makes 1 serving

Each Serving

Carb Servings
1

Exchanges
1/2 fat-free milk
1 fruit—with artificial
    sweetener 1/2

Nutrient analysis
calories 100—with
    artificial sweetener 85
total fat 1g
saturated fat 1g
cholesterol 5mg
sodium 129mg
total carbohydrate 18g—
    with artificial sweetener
    14g
dietary fiber 2g
sugars 17g—with artificial
    sweetener 13g
protein 5g

Buttermilk Fruit Shake

1/2 cup low-fat buttermilk
1/2 cup sliced fruit
1/4 teaspoon vanilla extract
2 ice cubes
sweetener to taste: 1–2 teaspoons sugar or the equivalent
    in artificial sweetener

Blend the first four ingredients until smooth.
Sweeten to taste.

Appetizers

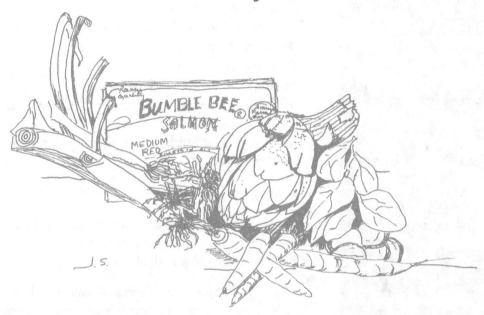

Keep calories and fat within reasonable limits by using fat-free sour cream and fat-free yogurt in recipes. Using vegetables for dipping will add fiber and keep the calories low.

Great for a party! Serve with raw vegetables such as cucumber slices, carrot sticks, and celery. This is also good when spread on small slices of whole-grain bread and broiled.

Makes 3 cups
12 servings

Each Serving
1/4 cup

Carb Servings
0

Exchanges
1 vegetable
1 fat

Nutrient Analysis
calories 70
total fat 4g
saturated fat 1g
cholesterol 6mg
sodium 182mg
total carbohydrate 4g
dietary fiber 2g
sugars 1g
protein 3g

Hot Artichoke and Spinach Dip

1/2 cup light mayonnaise
1/2 cup fat-free plain yogurt
1/2 cup grated Parmesan cheese
2 teaspoons dried or 3 tablespoons fresh minced onion
1 teaspoon chopped garlic
1/2 teaspoon dried basil
1/8 teaspoon ground black pepper
1 package (10 ounces) frozen chopped spinach, thawed, drained, and squeezed
1 can (14 ounces) artichoke hearts, drained, rinsed, and coarsely chopped

Preheat oven to 350 degrees.

Mix together mayonnaise, yogurt, Parmesan cheese, onion, garlic, basil, and pepper. Add spinach and artichoke hearts. Mix until blended.

Spread evenly in a pie plate that has been sprayed with nonstick cooking spray.

Bake for 25 minutes or until heated throughout.

Spinach Dip

1 package (10 ounces) frozen chopped spinach
.1/4 package (2 tablespoons) dry vegetable soup mix
1 3/4 cups fat-free plain yogurt
1 can (8 ounces) sliced water chestnuts, drained
   and chopped
1/4 cup light mayonnaise
2 tablespoons chopped green onion
1/4 teaspoon ground mustard

Thaw spinach, drain, and squeeze until dry. Stir dry soup before measuring to mix evenly.

Combine all ingredients and mix well. Chill and serve with raw vegetables or slices of whole-grain bread.

NOTE: Cube the bread that you remove and use it to spread the dip on.

This is a low-calorie version of a favorite hors d'oeuvre. It looks impressive if you hollow a round loaf of whole-grain bread and fill it with the dip.

Makes 3 1/2 cups
14 servings

Each Serving
1/4 cup

Carb Servings
0

Exchanges
1 vegetable
1/2 fat

Nutrient Analysis
calories 42
total fat 2g
saturated fat 0g
cholesterol 2mg
sodium 87mg
total carbohydrate 5g
dietary fiber 1g
sugars 3g
protein 2g

This is a delicious spread that even children like. Liquid smoke gives a special flavor, but it can be omitted. Red canned salmon or leftover fresh salmon work the best in this recipe.

Makes about 3 cups
24 servings

Each Serving
2 tablespoons

Carb Servings
0

Exchanges
1 lean meat

Nutrient Analysis
calories 38
total fat 1g
saturated fat 0g
cholesterol 6mg
sodium 158mg
total carbohydrate 1g
dietary fiber 0g
sugars 1g
protein 5g

Smoked Salmon Spread

1 tub (12 ounces) fat-free cream cheese
1/2 cup fat-free sour cream
1 tablespoon lemon juice
1 1/2 teaspoons Worcestershire sauce
1 teaspoon hickory liquid smoke*
1/8 teaspoon salt (optional)
1/8 teaspoon ground black pepper
1 can (14.75 ounces) red salmon, drained, or 2 cups cooked and flaked fresh salmon
2 tablespoons chopped celery
2 tablespoons chopped green onion

Have cream cheese at room temperature.

Blend the first seven ingredients in a mixer.

Remove skin from salmon and mash bones, if using canned. Mix salmon, celery, and onion with the cream cheese mixture.

Spread on raw vegetables or whole-grain crackers.

*_Hickory liquid smoke can be found in the grocery store next to the barbecue sauce._

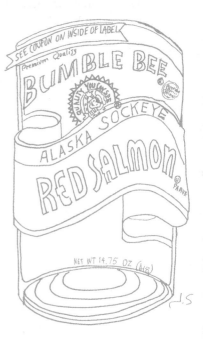

Chinese Barbecued Pork

1 pound boneless pork tenderloin (2 inches wide)
1/2 cup Chinese barbecue sauce
2 tablespoons ground mustard or bottled hot mustard

Marinate pork in barbecue sauce overnight (or at least 4 hours) in refrigerator. Discard marinade.

Preheat oven to 350 degrees. Roast meat for 30 minutes or until meat juices run clear.

Slice 1/8- to 1/4-inch thick and serve hot or refrigerate and serve cold.

To make hot mustard sauce from ground mustard:
Mix 2 tablespoons of ground mustard with an equal amount of cold water. Stir until the consistency of thick cream.

Allow to set 10 minutes to develop full flavor.

To serve: Dip pork in hot mustard sauce.

This is as good as the barbecued pork you order as an appetizer in Chinese restaurants. You can also serve this as a main dish by increasing the serving to 3 ounces.

Makes 16 Servings
32 slices

Each Serving
2 slices (1 ounce)

Carb Servings
0

Exchanges
1 lean meat

Nutrient Analysis
calories 47
total fat 2g
saturated fat 0g
cholesterol 16mg
sodium 42mg
total carbohydrate 2g
dietary fiber 0g
sugars 1g
protein 7g

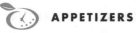

This is great on baked potatoes or can be used as a dip for vegetables. It is far more flavorful than sour cream. The addition of chopped green onion is also good.

Makes 1 1/4 cups
12 servings

Each Serving
2 tablespoons

Carb Servings
0

Exchanges
free

Nutrient Analysis
calories 15
total fat 0g
saturated fat 0g
cholesterol 1mg
sodium 79mg
total carbohydrate 1g
dietary fiber 0g
sugars 1g
protein 3g

Cottage Cheese Dip and Topping

1 cup low-fat cottage cheese
1/4 cup fat-free milk

Place all ingredients in blender. Process on high speed until smooth and creamy.

VARIATION: *Dill Cottage Cheese Dip*–Add 1 teaspoon of dried dill weed to mixture when blending.

Creamy Seafood Dip

4 ounces fat-free cream cheese
2 cups low-fat cottage cheese
3 tablespoons lemon juice
2 teaspoons prepared horseradish
1/4 teaspoon Tabasco sauce
1/4 cup chopped green onion
1 can (6.5 ounces) minced clams, shrimp, or crab, drained
    and rinsed

Have cream cheese at room temperature.

In a blender or food processor, mix cheeses with the next
three ingredients until smooth. Stir in onions and seafood.
Serve with raw vegetables or whole-grain crackers.

VARIATION: *Smoky Seafood Dip*–Add 1 teaspoon of hickory
liquid smoke when blending ingredients.

*This is a good choice for
a party. Fresh shrimp or
crab can be used in place
of canned.*

Makes 3 cups
24 servings

Each Serving
2 tablespoons

Carb Servings
0

Exchanges
Free

Nutrient Analysis
calories 22
total fat 0g
saturated fat 0g
cholesterol 2mg
sodium 116mg
total carbohydrate 1g
dietary fiber 0g
sugars 1g
protein 4g

Refrigerator Bran Muffins

1 cup All-Bran cereal
1 cup boiling water
2 cups low-fat buttermilk
1 1/4 cups sugar
1/2 cup egg substitute (equal to 2 eggs)
1/2 cup canola oil
1 1/2 cups whole-wheat flour
1 cup unbleached all-purpose flour
2 1/2 teaspoons baking soda
1/2 teaspoon salt (optional)
1 cup dried fruit (optional)
2 cups Bran Buds or 100% Bran cereal

In a small bowl, pour boiling water over the All-Bran cereal and let stand until softened.

In a large bowl, mix buttermilk, sugar, egg substitute, and oil. Add the All-Bran/water mixture to the egg mixture.

Mix the flours, baking soda, and salt in a small bowl. Stir into the egg mixture and mix just until moistened. If using dried fruit, add now. Stir in Bran Buds or 100% Bran cereal.

Follow directions below for microwave or conventional oven.

CONVENTIONAL OVEN: Preheat oven to 375 degrees. Pour about 1/4 cup batter into muffin tins sprayed with nonstick cooking spray or tins lined with cupcake papers. Bake for 15 minutes (20 minutes for chilled batter).

MICROWAVE OVEN: For one muffin: Pour 1/4 cup batter into cupcake paper. Cook on high 55–70 seconds, rotating 1/4 turn halfway through cooking.

NOTE: One serving is a good source of fiber.

Make this recipe to have on hand for fresh-baked breakfast muffins. The batter can be covered and stored in the refrigerator for up to three weeks. These are lower in sugar and fat than most bran muffins.

Makes 28 muffins

Each Serving
1 muffin

Carb Servings
1 1/2

Exchanges
1 1/2 starch
1 fat

Nutrient Analysis
calories 141
total fat 5g
saturated fat 0g
cholesterol 1mg
sodium 188mg
total carbohydrate 25g
dietary fiber 4g
sugars 12g
protein 3g

Makes 24 servings

Each Serving

Carb Servings
1 1/2

Exchanges
1 1/2 starch
1 fat

Nutrient Analysis
calories 164
total fat 5g
saturated fat 0g
cholesterol 0mg
sodium 136mg
total carbohydrate 25g
dietary fiber 2g
sugars 9g
protein 4g

Applesauce Oatmeal Coffee Cake

3 cups oats (old fashioned or quick)
1 1/2 cups unbleached all-purpose flour
1 cup whole-wheat flour
1 cup firmly packed brown sugar
1 tablespoon baking powder
1 teaspoon ground allspice
1/2 teaspoon ground cinnamon
2 cups unsweetened applesauce
1 cup fat-free milk
1/2 cup canola oil
1/2 cup egg substitute (equal to 2 eggs)

Optional Topping:
2 tablespoons firmly packed brown sugar and 1/4 teaspoon ground cinnamon

Preheat oven to 375 degrees.

Combine the first eight ingredients in a large bowl.

Mix the next four ingredients in a small bowl. Add to the dry ingredients and stir just until moistened.

Pour into a 9-inch by 13-inch baking dish that has been sprayed with nonstick cooking spray. Sprinkle optional topping ingredients over batter. Bake for 35–40 minutes or until golden brown.

VARIATIONS: Make half of this recipe and bake in a 9-inch by 9-inch baking pan for 25–30 minutes.

Applesauce Oatmeal Muffins–For muffins, bake at 400 degrees for 15–20 minutes. The full recipe makes about 24 muffins.

Blueberry Coffee Cake

2 cups oats (old fashioned or quick)
1 2/3 cups unbleached all-purpose flour
1 cup whole-wheat flour
1 cup firmly packed brown sugar
1 tablespoon baking powder
1 teaspoon salt (optional)
1 teaspoon ground cinnamon
1/2 teaspoon ground cloves
2 cups fat-free milk
1/2 cup egg substitute (equal to 2 eggs)
1/2 cup canola oil
2 cups fresh or frozen blueberries

Optional Topping:
2 tablespoons firmly packed brown sugar and 1/4
teaspoon ground cinnamon

Preheat oven to 375 degrees.

Combine the first eight
ingredients in a large bowl.

Mix milk, egg, and oil in a small
bowl. Add to the dry ingredients and
mix just until moistened. Add blueberries. Pour
into a 9-inch by 13-inch baking pan that has been
sprayed with nonstick cooking spray.

Bake for 35–40 minutes or until golden brown.

VARIATIONS: Make half of this recipe and bake in a 9-inch by 9-inch baking pan for 25–30 minutes.

Blueberry Muffins–For muffins, bake at 425 degrees for 15–20 minutes. The full recipe makes about 24 muffins.

This large coffee cake is great for a brunch. It also freezes well. See the variations below for a smaller coffee cake or for making muffins. This is lower in sugar and fat than most coffee cakes.

Makes 24 servings

Each Serving

Carb Servings
1 1/2

Exchanges
1 1/2 starch
1 fat

Nutrient Analysis
calories 156
total fat 5g
saturated fat 0g
cholesterol 0mg
sodium 82mg
total carbohydrate 24g
dietary fiber 2g
sugars 8g
protein 4g

Makes 12 servings

Each Serving

Carb Servings
1

Exchanges
1 starch

Nutrient Analysis
calories 104
total fat 1g
saturated fat 0g
cholesterol 0mg
sodium 215mg
total carbohydrate 20g
dietary fiber 1g
sugars 1g
protein 3g

Italian Focaccia Bread

1 loaf (1 pound) whole-wheat Focaccia bread
1 teaspoon olive oil
1 teaspoon Italian seasoning
1 teaspoon grated Parmesan cheese

Preheat oven to 375 degrees.

Spread olive oil over top of bread. Sprinkle with Italian seasoning and cheese.

Bake for 20 minutes or until golden brown.

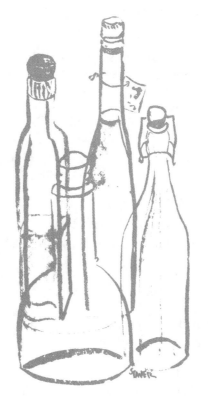

 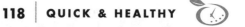

Gravies and Sauces

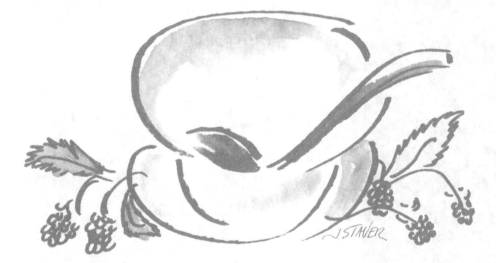

You'll find a few sauces in this section that will add interest to meals and satisfy your palate. Also included are fat-free gravies that taste great without the extra calories.

Spanish Yogurt Sauce

1 cup fat-free plain yogurt
1/2 cup salsa, thick and chunky
1 teaspoon dried parsley
1/2 teaspoon dried cilantro or 2 tablespoons chopped
   fresh cilantro
1/4 teaspoon ground cumin

Mix all ingredients and refrigerate
until serving.

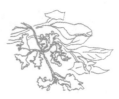

Thick and Chunky Salsa

1 can (14.5 ounces) diced tomatoes*
2 medium tomatoes, chopped (about 2 cups)
3 green onions, chopped (about 3/4 cup)
1/2 cup chopped fresh cilantro
1 can (4 ounces) diced green chiles
1 tablespoon chopped garlic
1/2 teaspoon salt (optional)
1/8 teaspoon ground black pepper

Combine all ingredients.

Serve with your favorite Mexican food or as a dip.

Sodium is figured for no added salt.

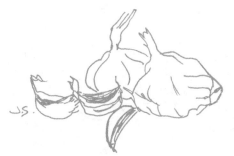

This is a great addition to any Mexican dish and can also be served over an omelet. The addition of cilantro makes this especially good.

Makes 4 cups
16 servings

Each Serving
1/4 cup

Carb Servings
0

Exchanges
free

Nutrient Analysis
calories 14
total fat 0g
saturated fat 0g
cholesterol 0mg
sodium 28mg
total carbohydrate 3g
dietary fiber 1g
sugars 2g
protein 1g

Serve this with the Oven-Fried Fish or the Oven-Fried Oysters recipe in this book. It's a good low-fat replacement for tartar sauce.

Makes 2 cups
8 servings

Each Serving
1/4 cup

Carb Servings
0

Exchanges
1/2 fat

Nutrient Analysis
calories 37
total fat 3g
saturated fat 1g
cholesterol 3mg
sodium 87mg
total carbohydrate 3g
dietary fiber 0g
sugars 1g
protein 1g

Fresh Cucumber Sauce for Seafood

1 cup chopped cucumber, not peeled
1/2 cup fat-free plain yogurt
1/4 cup chopped green onion
1/4 cup light mayonnaise
1 tablespoon lemon juice
1 teaspoon Dijon mustard
1 teaspoon dried minced onion or 1 tablespoon fresh
   minced onion
1/4 teaspoon salt (optional)

Combine all ingredients. Cover and chill before serving.

Serve cold with seafood.

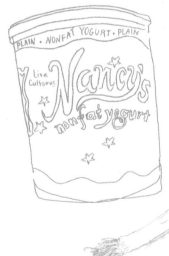

Fruit Sauce

1 1/2 cups fresh raspberries or sliced strawberries or one
    12-ounce package frozen raspberries or strawberries
4 teaspoons sugar or the equivalent in artificial sweetener
1 tablespoon lemon juice

FRESH FRUIT: Place 1/2 cup of fruit in a blender with
sweetener and lemon juice. Blend until smooth. Add
remaining fruit and stir into mixture.

FROZEN FRUIT: Thaw fruit. Place half of the fruit in
blender with sweetener and lemon juice. Blend until
smooth. Drain remaining fruit and stir into mixture.

NOTE: One serving is a good source of fiber.

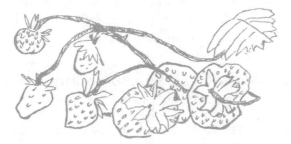

*This is great on pancakes
or as a sauce for cooked
and chilled asparagus.*

Makes 1 1/4 cups
5 servings

Each Serving
1/4 cup

Carb Servings
1/2—with artificial
    sweetener 0

Exchanges
1/2 fruit—free with
    artificial sweetener

Nutrient Analysis
calories 32—with artificial
    sweetener 19
total fat 0g
saturated fat 0g
cholesterol 0mg
sodium 1mg
total carbohydrate 8g—
    with artificial sweetener
    4g
dietary fiber 3g
sugars 5g—with artificial
    sweetener 2g
protein 0g

Flour Gravy

This will remind you of traditional gravy but it is so much lower in calories because it has no fat. You can use canned broth or instant bouillon mixed with water.

Makes 1 cup
8 servings

Each Serving
2 tablespoons

Carb Servings
0

Exchanges
free

Nutrient Analysis
calories 9
total fat 0g
saturated fat 0g
cholesterol 0mg
sodium 47mg
total carbohydrate 2g
dietary fiber 0g
sugars 0g
protein 1g

1 cup cold fat-free broth*, divided (chicken, turkey, or beef)
2 tablespoons unbleached all-purpose flour
seasonings to taste

Pour 1/4 cup of broth in a covered container. Add flour and shake well to prevent lumps.

Follow directions below for microwave or stovetop.

STOVETOP: In a small saucepan, combine remainder of broth with flour mixture. Cook on medium until boiling, while stirring constantly with a wire whisk. Continue stirring until thickened.

MICROWAVE OVEN: In a 4-cup glass measuring cup, combine remainder of broth with flour mixture. Heat on high for 2–3 minutes (stirring well with a wire whisk after each minute) or until thickened.

NOTE: Use 3 1/2 tablespoons of flour for one 14.5-ounce can of broth.

VARIATION: *Mushroom Gravy*—Add one small can of drained mushrooms after the gravy is thickened.

**Sodium is figured for reduced sodium.*

Cornstarch Gravy

1 cup cold fat-free broth*, divided (chicken, turkey, or beef)
1 tablespoon cornstarch
seasonings to taste

Pour 1/4 cup cold broth in a small container. Add cornstarch and mix well.

Follow directions below for microwave or stovetop.

STOVETOP: In a small saucepan, combine remainder of broth with cornstarch mixture. Cook on medium until boiling, while stirring constantly with a wire whisk. Continue stirring until thickened.

MICROWAVE OVEN: In a 4-cup glass measuring cup, combine remainder of broth with cornstarch mixture. Heat on high for 2–3 minutes (stirring well with a wire whisk after each minute) or until thickened.

NOTE: Use 1 3/4 tablespoons cornstarch for one 14.5-ounce can of broth.

VARIATION: *Mushroom Gravy*—Add one small can of drained mushrooms after the gravy is thickened. For a thicker gravy, increase cornstarch to 1 1/2 tablespoons.

Sodium is figured for reduced sodium.

This gravy contains no fat. It is the consistency of sauces used in Chinese food and has a clearer appearance than a flour gravy. Canned broth works well in this recipe.

Makes 1 cup
8 servings

Each Serving
2 tablespoons

Carb Servings
0

Exchanges
free

Nutrient Analysis
calories 6
total fat 0g
saturated fat 0g
cholesterol 0mg
sodium 47mg
total carbohydrate 1g
dietary fiber 0g
sugars 0g
protein 0g

Soups and Stews

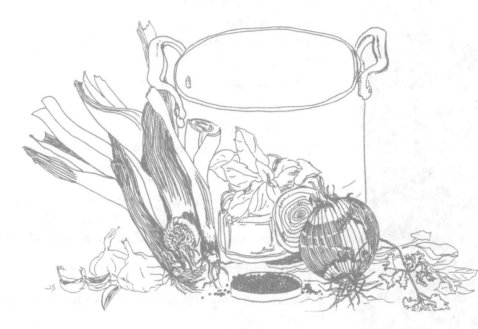

Soups are great on a cold winter day. Several of these recipes make a large amount, so plan on leftovers or freeze for later use. Freezing in one-cup containers makes a perfect choice for lunch. Many of these recipes are high in fiber.

Makes 8 cups
5 servings

Each Serving
1 1/2 cups

Carb Servings
1

Exchanges
3 vegetable
1/2 fat

Nutrient Analysis
calories 91
total fat 3g
saturated fat 0g
cholesterol 0mg
sodium 22mg
total carbohydrate 16g
dietary fiber 3g
sugars 10g
protein 3g

Gazpacho

1 large cucumber, not peeled, quartered
2 medium tomatoes, quartered
1 green bell pepper, quartered
1 medium onion, quartered
3 cups tomato juice,* divided
1 tablespoon olive oil
1 tablespoon lemon juice
1 teaspoon chopped garlic
1/2 teaspoon hot pepper sauce (optional)
1/4 teaspoon salt (optional)
1/4 teaspoon ground black pepper
dash cayenne pepper

Optional Toppings:
1/2–1 cup chopped fresh cilantro
fat-free sour cream or fat-free plain yogurt

In a blender or food processor, combine the cucumber, tomato, green pepper, onion, and 1 1/2 cups of the tomato juice. Process the ingredients until mixture is still chunky.

Mix in remaining ingredients. Chill thoroughly.

Serve in small bowls topped with cilantro and sour cream or yogurt.

NOTE: One serving is a good source of fiber.

Sodium is figured for no added salt.

 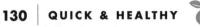

Vegetable Soup

1 can (14.5 ounces) fat-free broth* (chicken or beef)
1 1/2 cups sliced vegetables, any combination of:
cabbage, broccoli, carrots, onions, zucchini, celery,
tomatoes, cauliflower, mushrooms

Follow directions below for microwave or stovetop.

STOVETOP: Mix all ingredients in a small saucepan. Cover
and simmer for 10–15 minutes or until vegetables are
tender.

MICROWAVE OVEN: Mix all ingredients in a 1-quart glass
bowl. Cover and cook on high for about 5–10 minutes
(stir twice during cooking) until vegetables are tender.

*Sodium is figured for reduced sodium.

*Fresh shredded cabbage
is especially good in this
soup, but any vegetable
will do. Add cubed
chicken breast and cook
with the vegetables for a
more hearty soup.*

Makes 2 1/2 cups
2 servings

Each Serving
1 1/4 cups

Carb Servings
1/2

Exchanges
1 vegetable

Nutrient Analysis
calories 36
total fat 0g
saturated fat 0g
cholesterol 0mg
sodium 367mg
total carbohydrate 6g
dietary fiber 2g
sugars 3g
protein 3g

This simple and tasty soup can be made with canned, frozen, or fresh shrimp. Thaw frozen shrimp before serving.

Makes 1 1/2 cups
1 serving

Each Serving

Carb Servings
1

Exchanges
2 vegetable
2 lean meat

Nutrient Analysis
calories 129
total fat 1g
saturated fat 0g
cholesterol 166mg
sodium 235mg
total carbohydrate 11g
dietary fiber 1g
sugars 9g
protein 20g

Chilled Tomato-Shrimp Soup

1 cup tomato juice*
1/2 cup (3 ounces) cooked and cleaned shrimp
1/2 tablespoon lemon juice
1/2 teaspoon prepared horseradish
1/8 teaspoon Worcestershire sauce
1 drop Tabasco sauce

Combine all ingredients. Chill before serving.

Sodium is figured for no added salt.

 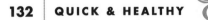

Italian Cioppino

1 can (28 ounces) diced tomatoes*, not drained
1 can (8 ounces) tomato sauce*
1 cup chopped onion
1/2 cup fat-free chicken broth* or white wine
1 tablespoon dried parsley
2 teaspoons chopped garlic
1 teaspoon each: dried basil, dried thyme, dried
    marjoram, and dried oregano
1 bay leaf
1/4 teaspoon ground black pepper
1 pound fish fillets (or cleaned shrimp, clams, crab)

Add all ingredients, except fish, in a medium saucepan.
Simmer for 20–30 minutes, stirring occasionally.

Meanwhile, cut fish into 1/2-inch
chunks. Add fish to saucepan
and cook 10 minutes or until
done. Discard bay leaf before
serving.

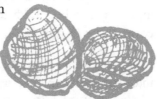

NOTE: One serving is a good source of fiber.

COOKING TIP: Use a combination of seafood such as
shrimp, clams, and crab. If uncooked, add with the fish. If
using precooked seafood, just add to heat.

VARIATION: *Italian Cioppino with Zucchini*—Add 2 cups
sliced zucchini before simmering.

Sodium is figured for no added salt/reduced sodium.

*I like the flavor of this
seafood stew. Don't limit
yourself to just fish, since
shrimp, clams, and crab
also taste good in this dish.*

Makes 6 cups
4 servings

Each Serving
1 1/2 cups

Carb Servings
1 1/2

Exchanges
4 vegetable
3 lean meat

Nutrient Analysis
calories 207
total fat 2g
saturated fat 0g
cholesterol 43mg
sodium 169mg
total carbohydrate 22g
dietary fiber 4g
sugars 13g
protein 27g

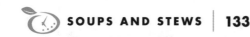

This low-calorie version of chowder has an excellent flavor.

Makes 6 cups
4 servings

Each Serving
1 1/2 cups

Carb Servings
1 1/2

Exchanges
1 starch
1/2 fat-free milk
2 lean meat

Nutrient Analysis
calories 220
total fat 2g
saturated fat 0g
cholesterol 43mg
sodium 156mg
total carbohydrate 22g
dietary fiber 2g
sugars 8g
protein 28g

New England Fish Chowder

1 1/2 cups diced new potatoes
1 cup water
1/2 cup chopped green pepper
1/2 cup chopped onion
1/2 teaspoon dried thyme
2 tablespoons cornstarch
2 cups fat-free milk
1/2 teaspoon salt (optional)
1/8 teaspoon ground black pepper
3/4 pound fish fillets, cut into 1-inch pieces
1/4 pound scallops (fish can be substituted)

In a medium saucepan, combine the first five ingredients and bring to a boil. Reduce heat to low and simmer, covered, for 15 minutes or until potatoes are tender.

Mix cornstarch with milk and remaining seasonings. Stir into soup and bring to a boil, stirring constantly until slightly thickened. Reduce heat and add seafood. Simmer until seafood is cooked.

Thai Chicken Soup

1 pound skinless, boneless chicken breasts, cut into
    bite-size pieces
4 cups fat-free chicken broth*
2 cups water
2 cups bite-size broccoli pieces
2 cups snow pea pods, cut in half (about 6 ounces)
2 cups chopped red bell pepper
6 ounces uncooked angel hair pasta, broken into
    small pieces
2 tablespoons minced fresh ginger
1 tablespoon chopped garlic
1 tablespoon lite soy sauce
1 teaspoon ground cumin
1/2–1 teaspoon ground fresh chili paste** (optional)
1/2 cup chopped fresh cilantro (optional)

In a large saucepan that has been sprayed with nonstick
cooking spray, sauté chicken for a few minutes. Add
remaining ingredients, except cilantro. Bring to a boil.

Reduce heat to low. Cover and simmer for 10–15 minutes
or until noodles are cooked and vegetables are tender.
Serve topped with fresh cilantro.

NOTE: One serving is a good source of fiber.

Sodium is figured for reduced sodium.

**Found in the Asian section of the grocery store.*

This soup gets a unique flavor from the fresh ginger. If you like spicy-hot foods, add the fresh chili paste.

Makes 10 1/2 cups
6 servings

Each Serving
1 3/4 cups

Carb Servings
2

Exchanges
1 1/2 starch
1 vegetable
3 lean meat

Nutrient Analysis
calories 233
total fat 2g
saturated fat 0g
cholesterol 43mg
sodium 406mg
total carbohydrate 28g
dietary fiber 3g
sugars 5g
protein 25g

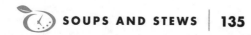

Makes 6 cups
6 servings

Each Serving
1 cup

Carb Servings
1

Exchanges
1/2 starch
1 vegetable

Nutrient Analysis
calories 79
total fat 1g
saturated fat 0g
cholesterol 0mg
sodium 326mg
total carbohydrate 14g
dietary fiber 1g
sugars 2g
protein 5g

Oriental Noodle Soup

5 cups fat-free chicken broth*
3/4 teaspoon garlic powder
1/4 teaspoon ground black pepper
3 ounces uncooked angel hair pasta
4 green onions, sliced thin
3/4 cup thinly sliced mushrooms
1/2 cup thinly sliced carrots

Combine the first three ingredients in a medium stockpot. Bring to a boil.

Break pasta into small pieces. Add pasta and vegetables to the stockpot.

Cook for 5–6 minutes or until pasta is tender.

Sodium is figured for reduced sodium.

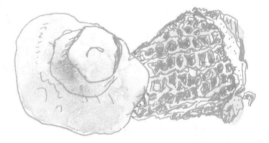

Taco Soup

1 pound extra lean ground beef or ground turkey (7% fat)
1 medium onion, chopped
2 cans (15 ounces each) pinto or chili beans, drained and rinsed
2 cans (8 ounces each) tomato sauce*
2 cans (14.5 ounces each) diced tomatoes*, not drained
1 cup water
1/2 package taco seasoning

Brown meat with onion in a stockpot that has been sprayed with nonstick cooking spray.

Add remaining ingredients and simmer for 30 minutes.

NOTE: One serving is an excellent source of fiber.

*Sodium is figured for no added salt.

**Half of the grams of fiber have been subtracted from the grams of total carbohydrate when figuring Carb Servings and Exchanges.*

This makes a large amount, so plan on freezing leftovers in lunch-size portions. This can be served with a dollop of fat-free yogurt or fat-free sour cream.

Makes 2 1/2 quarts
6 servings

Each Serving
1 1/2 cups

Carb Servings**
2

Exchanges**
1 1/2 starch
3 vegetable
2 lean meat

Nutrient Analysis
calories 285
total fat 6g
saturated fat 2g
cholesterol 48mg
sodium 271mg
total carbohydrate 40g
dietary fiber 10g
sugars 11g
protein 23g

The ingredients may seem a bit unusual but they combine to make a wonderfully unique flavor. This is a simple meal that you can complete with a salad. Add more curry if you like spicy foods.

Makes 8 cups
4 servings

Each Serving
2 cups

Carb Servings
1 1/2

Exchanges
1 starch
1/2 fruit
3 lean meat

Nutrient Analysis
calories 248
total fat 2g
saturated fat 0g
cholesterol 65mg
sodium 456mg
total carbohydrate 24g
dietary fiber 2g
sugars 6g
protein 31g

Chicken Curry Soup

1 pound skinless, boneless chicken breasts, cut into bite-size pieces
4 cups fat-free chicken broth*
2/3 cup uncooked quick-cooking brown rice
1 medium apple, peeled and diced (about 1 1/2 cups)
1/2 cup chopped onion
1 1/2 teaspoons curry powder
1/2 teaspoon salt (optional)
1/4 teaspoon ground black pepper
3 tablespoons unbleached all-purpose flour
1 cup water

In a large saucepan, sauté chicken for 3 minutes. Add chicken broth, rice, apple, onion, curry, salt, and pepper. Bring to a boil. Reduce heat to low. Cover and simmer for 10 minutes.

Meanwhile, in a covered container, combine water and flour. Shake well to prevent lumps. Stir into hot soup. Bring to a boil, stirring constantly for 1 minute or until slightly thickened.

Sodium is figured for reduced sodium.

Minestrone Soup

1/3 cup each: dried green split peas, dried lentils, and pearl barley

1/2 cup dried black-eyed peas

4 1/2 cups water

3 1/2 cups fat-free beef broth*

2 1/2 cups chopped vegetables of your choice: celery, onion, zucchini, carrots, green pepper, mushrooms, etc.

1 can (14.5 ounces) diced tomatoes*, not drained

2 teaspoons dried basil

1 1/2 teaspoons dried oregano

1 teaspoon salt (optional)

1 teaspoon chopped garlic

1/2 teaspoon ground black pepper

2 bay leaves

3 tablespoons grated Parmesan cheese

Wash peas, lentils, and barley. Mix with water and broth in a large kettle.

Bring to a boil. Reduce heat, cover, and simmer for 30 minutes. Add remaining ingredients and simmer another hour or until peas are tender. Discard bay leaves.

Serve sprinkled with Parmesan cheese.

NOTE: One serving is an excellent source of fiber.

*Sodium is figured for reduced sodium/no added salt.

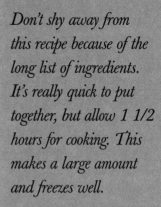

Don't shy away from this recipe because of the long list of ingredients. It's really quick to put together, but allow 1 1/2 hours for cooking. This makes a large amount and freezes well.

Makes 2 1/2 quarts
10 servings

Each Serving
1 cup

Carb Servings
1

Exchanges
1 starch
1 vegetable

Nutrient Analysis
calories 110
total fat 1g
saturated fat 0g
cholesterol 1mg
sodium 180mg
total carbohydrate 20g
dietary fiber 5g
sugars 4g
protein 6g

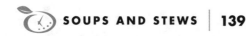

Makes 3 quarts
12 servings

Each Serving
1 cup

Carb Servings**
1 1/2

Exchanges**
1 starch
1 vegetable

Nutrient Analysis
calories 124
total fat 1g
saturated fat 0g
cholesterol 0mg
sodium 125mg
total carbohydrate 25g
dietary fiber 8g
sugars 7g
protein 7g

Three-Bean Soup

3 cups water
1 can (28 ounces) diced tomatoes,* not drained
1 can (15 ounces) kidney beans, drained and rinsed
1 can (15 ounces) black-eyed peas, drained and rinsed
1 can (15 ounces) garbanzo beans, drained and rinsed
1 can (6 ounces) tomato paste*
1 tablespoon Dijon mustard
1 1/2 teaspoons chopped garlic
1 teaspoon chili powder
1 teaspoon dried basil
1 teaspoon dried oregano
1/2 teaspoon ground cumin
1/2 teaspoon ground black pepper
1 1/3 cups frozen whole-kernel corn
1 cup chopped carrots
1 cup chopped zucchini or celery
1 medium onion, chopped

Combine the first 13 ingredients in a large stockpot.

Bring to a boil. Reduce heat and simmer, covered, for 10 minutes.

Stir in remaining vegetables and simmer, covered, for an additional 10 minutes.

NOTE: One serving is an excellent source of fiber.

Sodium is figured for no added salt.

**Half of the grams of fiber have been subtracted from the grams of total carbohydrate when figuring Carb Servings and Exchanges.*

Sausage and Bean Soup

1 package (16 ounces) low-fat turkey smoked sausage
1 medium onion chopped
4 cans (about 15 ounces each) of beans of your choice,
    drained and rinsed, Beans that work well are: black,
    kidney, pinto, garbanzo, lima
1 can (14.5 ounces) diced tomatoes*, not drained
2 cups fat-free chicken broth*
2 cups water
1 can (4 ounces) diced green chiles
1/2 cup salsa, thick and chunky
1 cup chopped fresh cilantro

Cut sausage into bite-size pieces.

In a large kettle, combine all ingredients except the
cilantro. Bring to a boil. Reduce heat to low. Cover and
simmer for 10 minutes.

Serve topped with cilantro.

NOTE: One serving is an excellent source of fiber.

This recipe is higher in sodium and should be limited by
those on a low-sodium diet.

Sodium is figured for no added salt/reduced sodium.

**Half of the grams of fiber have been subtracted from the grams of
total carbohydrate when figuring Carb Servings and Exchanges.*

*This is a meal in a bowl
and the best part is that
it can be prepared in
minutes. This makes a
large amount, so plan on
leftovers. We especially
like the spicy flavor and
the fresh cilantro.*

Makes 12 cups
8 servings

Each Serving
1 1/2 cups

Carb Servings**
2

Exchanges**
2 starch
1 vegetable
2 lean meat

Nutrient Analysis
calories 261
total fat 6g
saturated fat 2g
cholesterol 35mg
sodium 877mg
total carbohydrate 38g
dietary fiber 12g
sugars 8g
protein 19g

This is a great dish for a party because it really makes a large amount and it tastes so good. I also recommend freezing leftovers in 1-cup containers to have handy for lunch.

Makes 3 quarts
12 servings

Each Serving
1 cup

Carb Servings**
1 1/2

Exchanges**
1 starch
1 vegetable
3 lean meat

Nutrient Analysis
calories 242
total fat 6g
saturated fat 2g
cholesterol 47mg
sodium 141mg
total carbohydrate 27g
dietary fiber 11g
sugars 7g
protein 22g

Chili Con Carne

2 pounds extra-lean ground beef or ground turkey (7% fat)
3 cans (15 ounces each) kidney beans, drained and rinsed
1 can (28 ounces) diced tomatoes,* not drained
2 cans (8 ounces each) tomato sauce*
2 large onions, chopped
2 medium green peppers, chopped
2 tablespoons chili powder
1/4 teaspoon paprika
2 bay leaves

Brown the ground meat in a large kettle that has been sprayed with nonstick cooking spray. Add remaining ingredients.

Cover and simmer for 1 hour. Discard bay leaves before serving.

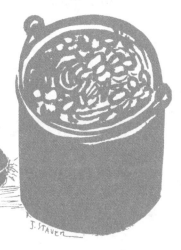

NOTE: One serving is an excellent source of fiber.

**Sodium is figured for no added salt.*

***Half of the grams of fiber have been subtracted from the grams of total carbohydrate when figuring Carb Servings and Exchanges.*

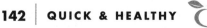

Tortilla Soup

1/2 pound skinless, boneless chicken breasts, cut into bite-size pieces
3 1/2 cups fat-free chicken broth*
1 can (15 ounces) black beans, drained and rinsed
1 1/3 cups frozen whole-kernel corn
1 can (14.5 ounces) diced tomatoes*, not drained
1 can (4 ounces) diced green chiles
3 corn tortillas (6-inch), cut in eighths

In a medium saucepan, sauté chicken for 3 minutes.

Add broth, beans, corn, tomatoes, and chiles. Simmer for 10 minutes. Add tortillas and simmer for an additional 10 minutes.

NOTE: One serving is an excellent source of fiber.

Sodium is figured for no added salt/reduced sodium.

**Half of the grams of fiber have been subtracted from the grams of total carbohydrate when figuring Carb Servings and Exchanges.*

This flavorful soup can be prepared in minutes. It will be enjoyed by all ages.

Makes 8 cups
4 servings

Each Serving
2 cups

Carb Servings**
2

Exchanges**
2 starch
1 vegetable
2 lean meat

Nutrient Analysis
calories 241
total fat 3g
saturated fat 0g
cholesterol 32mg
sodium 575mg
total carbohydrate 37g
dietary fiber 7g
sugars 9g
protein 24g

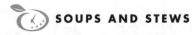

Vegetables

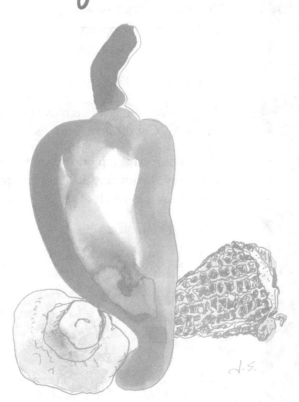

Recipes in this section include hot and cold vegetable dishes that work well with almost any meal. When preparing fresh vegetables, cook in the microwave or steam just until crisp-tender.

The rosemary gives a good flavor to these larger mushrooms without adding unwanted calories. Serve as an appetizer or as a side dish with chicken or beef.

Makes 4 servings

Each Serving

Carb Servings
0

Exchanges
1 vegetable

Nutrient Analysis
calories 32
total fat 1g
saturated fat 0mg
total cholesterol 0mg
sodium 5mg
total carbohydrate 4g
dietary fiber 1g
sugars 2g
protein 2g

Baked Portobello Mushrooms

4 Portobello mushrooms
1 teaspoon olive oil
1/4 teaspoon dried rosemary
1/8 teaspoon salt (optional)
dash ground black pepper

Preheat oven to 350 degrees.

Using a teaspoon, gently remove the gills (black underside). Cut off stems and discard.

Place mushrooms, top side up, on a baking sheet that has been sprayed with nonstick cooking spray. Brush with olive oil. Sprinkle with rosemary, salt, and pepper.

Bake for 10 minutes.

Roasted Eggplant Medley

1 small eggplant, not peeled (about 12–14 ounces), cut into 1-inch cubes (about 4 cups)

1 onion, cut in eighths

1 cup chopped bell pepper, green or yellow

1 tablespoon chopped garlic

1 teaspoon Italian seasoning

1/2 teaspoon salt (optional)

1/4 teaspoon ground black pepper

2 medium tomatoes, chopped (about 2 cups)

Preheat oven to 400 degrees.

In a large bowl, mix vegetables, except tomatoes, with garlic and seasonings.

Spread in a 9-inch by 13-inch baking pan that has been sprayed with nonstick cooking spray. Roast for 10–15 minutes.

Add tomatoes and return to oven for 5 minutes or until all vegetables are tender.

NOTE: One serving is a good source of fiber.

This is an attractive side dish that goes well with beef, fish, or chicken.

Makes 4 cups
8 servings

Each Serving
1/2 cup

Carb Servings
1/2

Exchanges
1 vegetable

Nutrient Analysis
calories 30
total fat 0g
saturated fat 0mg
cholesterol 0mg
sodium 4mg
total carbohydrate 7g
dietary fiber 3g
sugars 3g
protein 1g

Makes 3 1/2 cups
7 servings

Each Serving
1/2 cup

Carb Servings
1/2

Exchanges
1 vegetable

Nutrient Analysis
calories 29
total fat 0g
saturated fat 0mg
cholesterol 0mg
sodium 7mg
total carbohydrate 7g
dietary fiber 2g
sugars 3g
protein 1g

Zucchini, Tomato, and Onion

2 cups sliced onion
2 cups sliced tomato
2 cups sliced zucchini
1 1/2 teaspoons Italian seasoning
1/2 teaspoon salt (optional)
dash of ground black pepper

Preheat oven to 350 degrees.

Layer onion, tomato, and zucchini in a 2-quart casserole dish that has been sprayed with nonstick cooking spray.

Sprinkle each layer with seasonings.

Bake for 30–45 minutes, or until vegetables are tender.

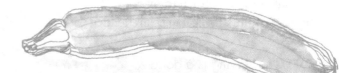

Basil Tomatoes

2 medium tomatoes, diced or sliced (about 2 cups)
1 teaspoon dried basil
1 teaspoon chopped garlic
1/2 teaspoon salt (optional)
1/8 teaspoon ground black pepper

Mix ingredients and let set at room temperature for at least 1 hour.

Serve plain or on a lettuce leaf.

One of my favorite recipes. The addition of basil gives an excellent flavor to fresh tomatoes.

Makes 2 cups
4 servings

Each Serving
1/2 cup

Carb Servings
0

Exchanges
free

Nutrient Analysis
calories 18
total fat 0g
saturated fat 0mg
cholesterol 0mg
sodium 5mg
total carbohydrate 4g
dietary fiber 1g
sugars 2g
protein 1g

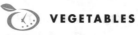

Makes 2 cups
4 servings

Each Serving
1/2 cup

Carb Servings
0

Exchanges
free

Nutrient Analysis
calories 19
total fat 0g
saturated fat 0mg
cholesterol 0mg
sodium 5mg
total carbohydrate 5g
dietary fiber 1g
sugars 3g
protein 1g

Italian Tomatoes

2 cups sliced tomatoes
1/4 cup red wine vinegar
1/4 teaspoon Italian seasoning
1/8 teaspoon ground black pepper
1/8 teaspoon garlic powder

Arrange tomatoes in a shallow bowl.

Mix remaining ingredients and pour over tomatoes.
Marinate 1/2 hour, at room temperature, before serving.

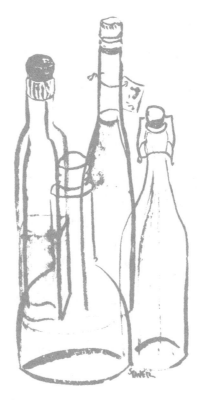

Gourmet Cucumbers

1/3 cup rice vinegar
1 tablespoon sugar or the equivalent in artificial
  sweetener
1 medium cucumber, not peeled, thinly sliced
  (about 2 cups)
1 cup sliced sweet onion
1/4 teaspoon ground black pepper
1/4 teaspoon dried dill weed (optional)

Mix vinegar with sugar. Add remaining ingredients.

Serve immediately or marinate in the refrigerator for
2 or 3 hours. Serve with a slotted spoon or drain liquid
before serving.

*This is a family favorite!
The rice vinegar that
you sweeten gives the
cucumbers an excellent
flavor.*

Makes 3 cups
6 servings

Each Serving
1/2 cup

Carb Servings
0

Exchanges
1 vegetable—free with
  artificial sweetener

Nutrient Analysis
calories 23—with artificial
  sweetener 14
total fat 0g
saturated fat 0mg
cholesterol 0mg
sodium 3mg
total carbohydrate 5g—
  with artificial sweetener
  3g
dietary fiber 0g
sugars 3g—with artificial
  sweetener 1g
protein 0g

You'll find this is a good substitute for a salad. This recipe can be prepared in advance and refrigerated for several days.

Makes 4 cups
8 servings

Each Serving
1/2 cup

Carb Servings
0

Exchanges
free

Nutrient Analysis
calories 19
total fat 1g
saturated fat 0mg
cholesterol 0mg
sodium 128mg
total carbohydrate 3g
dietary fiber 1g
sugars 2g
protein 1g

Marinated Vegetables

4 cups water
4 cups vegetables, cut into bite-size pieces, such as: broccoli, celery, green pepper, carrots, mushrooms, cauliflower, green beans
1/4 cup reduced-fat Italian dressing

Bring water to a boil. Add vegetables and return to a boil. Drain immediately and submerge in ice cold water. Drain.

Mix vegetables with Italian dressing and marinate in the refrigerator for 1 hour or until well chilled. Drain before serving.

Salsa Vegetables

1 cup chopped cucumber, not peeled
1 can (14.5 ounces) diced tomatoes* or 1 1/2 cups
   chopped fresh tomato
2/3 cup frozen whole-kernel corn
1/2 cup chopped bell pepper, red or green
1/4 cup chopped fresh cilantro
2 tablespoons red wine vinegar
1/2 teaspoon garlic powder
1/2 teaspoon ground cumin
1/4 teaspoon salt (optional)
1/8 teaspoon ground black pepper
1/8 teaspoon cayenne pepper

Combine ingredients and mix well. Serve cold.

Sodium is figured for no added salt.

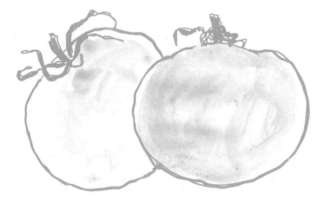

Serve this as a cold side dish with Mexican food. It is colorful and has a great flavor.

Makes 4 cups
8 servings

Each Serving
1/2 cup

Carb Servings
1/2

Exchanges
1 vegetable

Nutrient Analysis
calories 28
total fat 0g
saturated fat 0mg
cholesterol 0mg
sodium 10mg
total carbohydrate 6g
dietary fiber 1g
sugars 4g
protein 1g

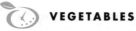

Seasoned Green Beans

This dish can be served either hot or cold. The rice vinegar and bacon bits add a good flavor to the beans.

1 tablespoon water
1 tablespoon dried or 1/4 cup fresh minced onion
1 can (14 ounces) green beans*, drained
1 tablespoon rice vinegar
2 teaspoons bacon-flavored soy bits
1/2 teaspoon sugar or the equivalent in artificial sweetener
1/4 teaspoon ground black pepper

Mix the first two ingredients in a medium bowl. Let set for 5–10 minutes.

Add remaining ingredients and mix well. Serve hot or cold.

Sodium is figured for no added salt.

Makes 4 servings
About 1 1/2 cups

Each Serving
About 1/3 cup

Carb Servings
1/2—with artificial sweetener 0

Exchanges
1 vegetable

Nutrient Analysis
calories 28—with artificial sweetener 26
total fat 0g
saturated fat 0mg
cholesterol 0mg
sodium 21mg
total carbohydrate 6g—with artificial sweetener 5g
dietary fiber 2g
sugars 2g—with artificial sweetener 1g
protein 1g

Salads

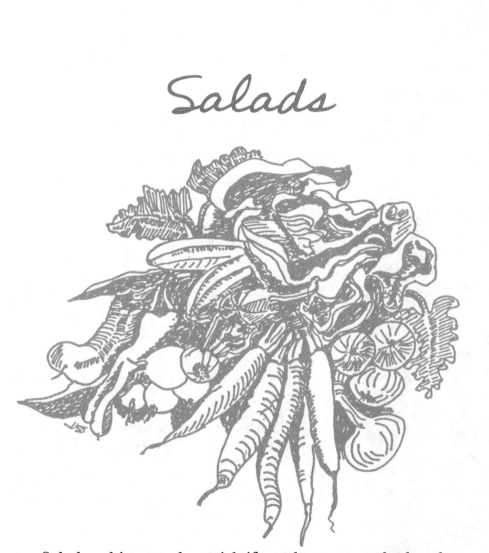

Salad making can be quick if you buy pre-washed and cut vegetables. Using a food processor also saves time, especially if you chop foods for several recipes at once. Salads in this section include main dishes, side dishes, and salads that can be served on a bed of lettuce or used as a sandwich spread.

Tangy grapefruit and mild avocado add variety to salad greens and make this a delicious and enjoyable salad.

Makes 10 cups
5 servings

Each Serving
2 cups

Carb Servings
1

Exchanges
1/2 fruit
1 vegetable
1 1/2 fat

Nutrient Analysis
calories 134—with
    artificial sweetener 128
total fat 8g
saturated fat 1g
cholesterol 0mg
sodium 30mg
total carbohydrate 16g—
    with artificial sweetener
    14g
dietary fiber 5g
sugars 10g—with artificial
    sweetener 8g
protein 3g

Grapefruit and Avocado Salad

1 medium avocado
2 tablespoons lime juice
1 grapefruit, peeled
1/2 cup thinly sliced green onions
10–12 ounces mixed salad greens (about 2 quarts), torn

Dressing:
2 tablespoons apple cider vinegar
1 tablespoon olive oil
1 tablespoon water
2 teaspoons sugar, or the equivalent in artificial sweetener
1/4 teaspoon ground cumin
1/8 teaspoon ground black pepper
1/8 teaspoon salt (optional)

Peel and slice the avocado. Pour lime juice over avocado to prevent browning.

Section grapefruit and cut into bite-size pieces. In a large salad bowl, mix grapefruit, green onion, and salad greens.

Drain avocado, reserving lime juice. Mix reserved lime juice with dressing ingredients. Add avocado to the salad. Pour dressing over salad and toss.

NOTE: One serving is an excellent source of fiber.

Most of the fat in this recipe is heart-healthy monounsaturated fat.

Pear Salad with Raspberry Dressing

2 medium pears, chopped, not peeled (about 3 cups)
1 tablespoon lemon juice
10–12 ounces mixed salad greens (about 2 quarts), torn
1/4 cup chopped walnuts or almonds
1/2 cup reduced-fat raspberry salad dressing

In a large salad bowl, mix chopped pears with lemon juice to prevent browning.

Add salad greens and nuts. Pour dressing over salad and toss.

NOTE: One serving is an excellent source of fiber.

Most of the fat in the recipe is heart-healthy omega-3 fat and polyunsaturated fat.

VARIATION: *Apple Salad with Raspberry Dressing*–Substitute chopped apples for the pears.

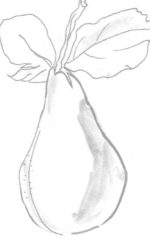

This is a great fall salad and will be popular with the whole family. The combination of fruit with nuts and raspberry dressing is pleasing to the palate.

Makes 10 cups
5 servings

Each Serving
2 cups

Carb Servings
1 1/2

Exchanges
1 fruit
2 vegetable
1 fat

Nutrient Analysis
calories 158
total fat 7g
saturated fat 0g
cholesterol 0mg
sodium 243mg
total carbohydrate 23g
dietary fiber 5g
sugars 15g
protein 3g

This is a refreshing salad that goes well with many dishes.

Makes 2 1/2 cups
5 servings

Each Serving
1/2 cup

Carb Servings
1/2

Exchanges
1/2 fruit

Nutrient Analysis
calories 39
total fat 0g
saturated fat 0g
cholesterol 0mg
sodium 51mg
total carbohydrate 8g
dietary fiber 1g
sugars 6g
protein 1g

Apple Salad Mold

1 small box (0.3 ounces) sugar-free cherry-flavored gelatin*
1 cup boiling water
1/2 cup apple juice
1/2 cup cold water
1 medium apple, not peeled, chopped (about 1 1/2 cups)
1/2 cup chopped celery

Dissolve gelatin in boiling water.

Combine juice and cold water. Add to gelatin and stir well. Refrigerate until slightly thickened. Add apple and celery. Mix well.

Refrigerate until set.

Any flavor of gelatin can be substituted.

Fruit Salad

4 cups sliced fruit
1 cup fruit-flavored fat-free, sugar-free yogurt

Mix fruit with yogurt in a
serving bowl.

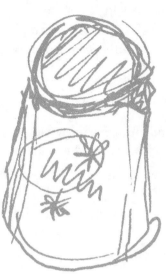

Makes 4 cups
8 servings

Each Serving
1/2 cup

Carb Servings
1

Exchanges
1 fruit

Nutrient Analysis
calories 60
total fat 0g
saturated fat 0g
cholesterol 1mg
sodium 23mg
total carbohydrate 14g
dietary fiber 1g
sugars 10g
protein 2g

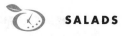

Makes 5 1/2 cups
7 servings

Each Serving
3/4 cup

Carb Servings
1

Exchanges
1/2 fruit
1/2 fat-free milk
1 lean meat

Nutrient Analysis
calories 121
total fat 1g
saturated fat 0g
cholesterol 3mg
sodium 328mg
total carbohydrate 16g
dietary fiber 0g
sugars 10g
protein 11g

Lime Cottage Salad

1 small box (0.3 ounces) sugar-free, lime-flavored gelatin
1 cup fat-free plain yogurt
2 cups low-fat, small-curd cottage cheese
1 can (20 ounces) crushed pineapple, in juice, drained
2 cups fat-free whipped topping

Mix gelatin with yogurt in a medium bowl. Add cottage cheese and pineapple. Mix well.

Gently mix in whipped topping. This is ready to serve or can be refrigerated for later use.

Romaine and Mandarin Orange Salad

1 medium avocado
1 tablespoon lime juice
10–12 ounces romaine lettuce (about 2 quarts), torn
2 cans (11 ounces each) mandarin oranges, in juice, drained

Dressing:
1/3 cup rice vinegar
1 tablespoon canola or sesame oil
1 1/2 tablespoons sugar or the equivalent in artificial sweetener
2 teaspoons lite soy sauce
2 teaspoons water
1/2 teaspoon ground ginger
1/2 teaspoon ground mustard
1/2 teaspoon salt (optional)
1/2 teaspoon ground black pepper

Peel and slice avocado. In a large salad bowl, pour lime juice over avocado to prevent browning. Add lettuce and mandarin oranges.

Mix dressing ingredients and shake well. Pour over salad ingredients and toss.

NOTE: One serving is a good source of fiber.

Most of the fat in this recipe is heart-healthy monounsaturated fat.

The sweet, tangy dressing makes this salad a standout. Also, consider using sesame oil, as it adds a unique flavor to this salad.

Makes 10 cups
5 servings

Each Serving
2 cups

Carb Servings
1

Exchanges
2 vegetable—with artificial sweetener 1
1/2 fruit
1 1/2 fat

Nutrient Analysis
calories 140—with artificial sweetener 125
total fat 8g
saturated fat 1g
cholesterol 0mg
sodium 112mg
total carbohydrate 17g—with artificial sweetener 13g
dietary fiber 4g
sugars 11g—with artificial sweetener 8g
protein 3g

 SALADS | 161

Makes 3 cups
4 servings

Each Serving
3/4 cup

Carb Servings
1/2

Exchanges
2 vegetable
1 fat

Nutrient Analysis
calories 97
total fat 7g
saturated fat 1g
cholesterol 0mg
sodium 11mg
total carbohydrate 10g
dietary fiber 4g
sugars 2g
protein 2g

Mexican Garden Salad

1 medium tomato, sliced and quartered (about 1 cup)
1 cup sliced cucumber, not peeled
1 cup chopped sweet onion
1 medium avocado, peeled and sliced
1/2 cup chopped fresh cilantro
1 tablespoon lime juice
1/4 teaspoon ground cumin
1/4 teaspoon salt (optional)
1/8 teaspoon ground black pepper

In a medium bowl, mix vegetables with remaining ingredients. Serve as is or on a bed of lettuce.

NOTE: One serving is a good source of fiber.

Most of the fat in this recipe is heart-healthy monounsaturated fat.

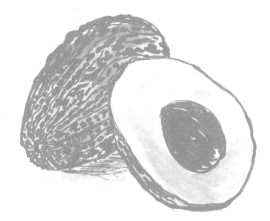

Italian Garden Salad

1 medium tomato, sliced and quartered (about 1 cup)
1 cup sliced cucumber, not peeled
1 cup chopped sweet onion
1 1/2 teaspoons dried basil
1 1/2 teaspoons chopped garlic
1/2 teaspoon salt (optional)
1/8 teaspoon ground black pepper

Combine all ingredients. Let set out for 30 minutes to 1 hour, at room temperature, before serving. Serve alone or on a lettuce leaf.

This salad is especially good when fresh vegetables are in season.

Makes 3 cups
4 servings

Each Serving
3/4 cup

Carb Servings
1/2

Exchanges
1 vegetable

Nutrient Analysis
calories 28
total fat 0g
saturated fat 0g
cholesterol 0mg
sodium 6mg
total carbohydrate 6g
dietary fiber 1g
sugars 2g
protein 1g

The red and yellow peppers add good flavor and color to this salad. It tastes best when marinated for several hours and is also great the next day.

Makes 8 cups
8 servings

Each Serving
1 cup

Carb Servings
0

Exchanges
1 vegetable

Nutrient Analysis
calories 33
total fat 0g
saturated fat 0g
cholesterol 0mg
sodium 227mg
total carbohydrate 5g
dietary fiber 1g
sugars 3g
protein 4g

Greek Salad

1 green pepper, sliced
1 red pepper, sliced
1 yellow pepper, sliced
1 cucumber, not peeled, sliced
3 tablespoons red wine vinegar
2 tablespoons lemon juice
1/4 teaspoon dried oregano
4 ounces fat-free feta cheese

Mix peppers and cucumber in a large bowl. Add vinegar, lemon juice, and oregano. Mix well. Cover and marinate for 15 minutes to several hours.

Toss well before serving and top with crumbled feta cheese.

 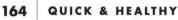

Broccoli Salad

4 cups broccoli florets
2 tomatoes, chopped (2 cups)
1 cup sliced mushrooms
4 teaspoons bacon-flavor soy bits

Dressing:
1/4 cup light mayonnaise
1 tablespoon dried parsley
1/4 teaspoon onion powder
1/8 teaspoon garlic powder

Mix vegetables and bacon bits in a medium bowl.

Make dressing by combining seasonings with mayonnaise.

Add dressing to vegetables and mix well.

NOTE: One serving is a good source of fiber.

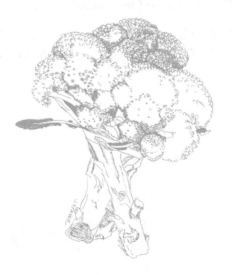

This makes a large amount so it is a good choice for a potluck. If you prefer the crunch of the soy bacon bits, add them just before serving.

Makes 6 cups
6 servings

Each Serving
1 cup

Carb Servings
1/2

Exchanges
1 vegetable
1 fat

Nutrient Analysis
calories 68
total fat 4g
saturated fat 1g
cholesterol 3mg
sodium 124mg
total carbohydrate 6g
dietary fiber 3g
sugars 3g
protein 3g

Keep these canned beans on hand so you can put together a salad in just a few minutes.

Makes 3 cups
6 servings

Each Serving
1/2 cup

Carb Servings*
1—with artificial
    sweetener 1/2

Exchanges*
1 starch—1/2 with
    artificial sweetener

Nutrient Analysis
calories 70—with artificial
    sweetener 62
total fat 1g
saturated fat 0g
cholesterol 0mg
sodium 40mg
total carbohydrate 15g—
    with artificial sweetener
    13g
dietary fiber 6g
sugars 4g—with artificial
    sweetener 2g
protein 4g

Three-Bean Salad

1/4 cup rice vinegar
1 tablespoon sugar or the equivalent in artificial
    sweetener
1 tablespoon dried or 1/4 cup fresh minced onion
1 can (14 ounces) green beans*, drained
1 can (8 ounces) garbanzo beans, drained and rinsed
1 can (8 ounces) kidney beans, drained and rinsed
1 tablespoon dried parsley
1/4 teaspoon onion powder
1/8 teaspoon garlic powder

In a medium bowl, combine vinegar, sugar, and onion.
Let set for 5 minutes.

Add beans and seasonings. Mix well. Drain before
serving.

NOTE: One serving is an excellent source of fiber.

*_Sodium is figured for no added salt._

**_Half of the grams of fiber have been subtracted from the grams of
total carbohydrate when figuring Carb Servings and Exchanges._

 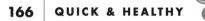

Cabbage Salad

6 cups chopped cabbage
3 green onions, chopped
3 tablespoons toasted sesame seeds

Dressing:
1/4 cup rice vinegar
1 tablespoon sugar or the equivalent in artificial
   sweetener

Mix the first three ingredients in a large bowl.

Combine rice vinegar with sugar. Add to cabbage and toss well.

This is ready to serve or you can refrigerate it for several hours before serving.

NOTE: One serving is a good source of fiber.

VARIATIONS: *Cabbage and Chicken Salad*–Just before serving, add 2 cups of cooked chicken.

Cabbage and Shrimp Salad–Just before serving, add 2 cups of cooked and cleaned shrimp. Frozen shrimp that has been thawed is preferred over canned.

To save time, use a food processor for chopping the cabbage. This is simple to prepare and has a good flavor.

Makes 6 cups
6 servings

Each Serving
1 cup

Carb Servings
1/2

Exchanges
2 vegetable

Nutrient Analysis
calories 54—with artificial
   sweetener 45
total fat 2g
saturated fat 0g
cholesterol 0mg
sodium 19mg
total carbohydrate 9g—
   with artificial sweetener
   7g
dietary fiber 3g
sugars 6g—with artificial
   sweetener 4g
protein 2g

This variation of the Three-Bean Salad uses fresh vegetables in place of some of the beans.

Makes 3 cups
6 servings

Each Serving
1/2 cup

Carb Servings
1—with artificial
    sweetener 1/2

Exchanges
1/2 starch
1 vegetable

Nutrient Analysis
calories 52—with artificial
    sweetener 44
total fat 0g
saturated fat 0g
cholesterol 0mg
sodium 28mg
total carbohydrate 11g—
    with artificial sweetener
    9g
dietary fiber 4g
sugars 4g—with artificial
    sweetener 2g
protein 3g

Vegetable Bean Salad

1/4 cup rice vinegar
1 tablespoon sugar or the equivalent in artificial
    sweetener
1 tablespoon dried or 1/4 cup fresh minced onion
1 can (8 ounces) green beans* or garbanzo beans,
    drained and rinsed
1 can (8 ounces) kidney beans, drained and rinsed
1 cup bite-size pieces of cauliflower or broccoli
1/2 cup sliced carrots
1 tablespoon dried parsley
1/4 teaspoon onion powder
1/8 teaspoon garlic powder

In a medium bowl, combine vinegar, sugar, and onion.

Let set for 5 minutes. Add vegetables and seasonings.
Mix well.

Drain before serving.

NOTE: One serving is a good source of fiber.

Sodium is figured for no added salt.

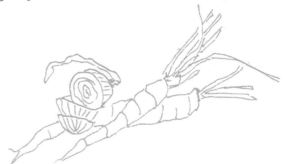

Macaroni Salad

8 ounces uncooked elbow macaroni
2 cups sliced celery
2 cups chopped red pepper
1/2 cup chopped green onion (optional)

Dressing:
1/2 cup light mayonnaise
1/3 cup rice vinegar
1 1/2 tablespoons sugar or the equivalent in artificial
    sweetener
1 tablespoon Dijon mustard
1/4 teaspoon ground black pepper

Cook macaroni according to package directions.
Drain and cool.

Prepare vegetables and place
in a large bowl.

In a small bowl, mix
dressing ingredients. Add
cooled macaroni and dressing to
vegetables. Toss well.

*The red pepper adds
color to this dish while
the rice vinegar and
mustard add a good
flavor. About half of this
recipe is vegetables.*

Makes 8 cups
10 servings

Each Serving
3/4 cup

Carb Servings
1 1/2—with artificial
    sweetener 1

Exchanges
1 starch
1 vegetable
1 fat

Nutrient Analysis
calories 141—with
    artificial sweetener 134
total fat 5g
saturated fat 1g
cholesterol 4mg
sodium 152mg
total carbohydrate 21g—
    with artificial sweetener
    19g
dietary fiber 2g
sugars 4g—with artificial
    sweetener 2g
protein 4g

The mustard and seasonings make this a tasty potato salad. Try using new red potatoes or Yukon gold.

Makes 6 servings
6 cups

Each Serving
1 cup

Carb Servings
1

Exchanges
1 starch

Nutrient Analysis
calories 74
total fat 1g
saturated fat 0g
cholesterol 1mg
sodium 78mg
total carbohydrate 14g
dietary fiber 2g
sugars 2g
protein 2g

Herb Potato Salad

1 pound thin-skinned new potatoes, not peeled (about 4 cups, cubed)
1 cup sliced celery
1/2 cup sliced green onion

Dressing:
3 tablespoons fat-free plain yogurt
1 tablespoon light mayonnaise
1 1/2 teaspoons Dijon mustard
1/2 teaspoon chopped garlic
1/2 teaspoon dried basil
1/4 teaspoon dried thyme
1/4 teaspoon onion powder
1/4 teaspoon salt (optional)

Cut potatoes in 1-inch cubes. Place in medium saucepan and cover with water. Bring to a boil. Cover, reduce heat, and simmer 12 minutes or until potatoes are tender. Drain.

Mix dressing ingredients.

Combine hot potatoes, celery, green onion, and dressing. Serve hot or refrigerate and serve cold.

Cinnamon Chicken Salad

The addition of cinnamon and cloves gives this chicken salad a unique taste.

Dressing:
2 tablespoons light mayonnaise
2 tablespoons fat-free plain yogurt
1/2 teaspoon ground cinnamon
1/8 teaspoon ground cloves
1/8 teaspoon ground black pepper
1/8 teaspoon salt (optional)

2 cups cooked and cubed chicken or turkey
1 cup seedless grapes
1/2 cup sliced celery
8 large lettuce leaves

Mix the dressing ingredients and set aside.

Combine chicken, grapes, and celery in a medium bowl.

Add dressing and toss. Serve on lettuce leaves.

Makes 4 cups
4 servings

Each Serving
1 cup

Carb Servings
1/2

Exchanges
1/2 fruit
3 lean meat

Nutrient Analysis
calories 169
total fat 5g
saturated fat 1g
cholesterol 57mg
sodium 125mg
total carbohydrate 10g
dietary fiber 1g
sugars 7g
protein 21g

Chinese Chicken Salad

This makes a large amount and is great for a potluck or a luncheon. Use a food processor to save time chopping.

Makes 14 cups
7 servings

Each Serving
2 cups

Carb Servings
1 1/2

Exchanges
1 starch
2 vegetable
1 lean meat
1/2 fat

Nutrient Analysis
calories 213—with
    artificial sweetener 209
total fat 6g
saturated fat 1g
cholesterol 31mg
sodium 262mg
total carbohydrate 24g—
    with artificial sweetener
    23g
dietary fiber 3g
sugars 4g
protein 15g

1 small head (1 1/2 pounds) Chinese Napa cabbage, shredded
2 cups cooked brown rice
2 cups cooked chicken, shredded
1 cup diagonally sliced celery
1/2 cup sliced green onion
1 can (16 ounces) bean sprouts, drained and rinsed
1 can (8 ounces) sliced water chestnuts, drained and chopped

Soy Dressing:
2 tablespoons canola oil
1/3 cup water
2–4 tablespoons lite soy sauce*
1 tablespoon cider vinegar
1 tablespoon catsup
1 tablespoon brown sugar or the equivalent in artificial sweetener
1/2 teaspoon ground ginger or 2 teaspoons fresh grated
1/4 teaspoon chopped garlic

In a large bowl, combine the first seven ingredients.

Prepare dressing by mixing ingredients in a covered container and shake to blend.

Toss dressing with salad up to 4 hours or just before serving. For an attractive presentation, save a few of the cabbage leaves to line a serving bowl.

Use the lesser amount of soy sauce if on a sodium-restricted diet.

NOTE: One serving is a good source of fiber.

Oriental Rice and Seafood Salad

2 cups cooked brown rice, cooled
1 pound cooked and cleaned salad shrimp
1 can (16 ounces) bean sprouts, drained and rinsed
2 stalks celery, diagonally sliced
1/2 cup chopped green pepper
2 green onions, thinly sliced
1 can (8 ounces) sliced water chestnuts, drained
1/4 cup rice vinegar
2 tablespoons lite soy sauce
1 tablespoon sugar or the equivalent in artificial
   sweetener

Combine the first seven ingredients in a large bowl.

Mix vinegar, soy sauce, and sugar. Pour over salad and mix well. Chill before serving.

NOTE: One serving is a good source of fiber.

VARIATION: *Oriental Rice and Chicken Salad*—Substitute 2 cups of cooked and cubed chicken for the shrimp.

This is a delicious recipe that makes enough for a crowd. I really like the flavor you get from the soy sauce and rice vinegar. Use quick-cooking brown rice to save time.

Makes 8 cups
5 servings

Each Serving
1 1/2 cups

Carb Servings
2

Exchanges
1 1/2 starch
1 vegetable
2 lean meat

Nutrient Analysis
calories 235—with
   artificial sweetener 225
total fat 2g
saturated fat 0g
cholesterol 175mg
sodium 483mg
total carbohydrate 30g—
   with artificial sweetener
   28g
dietary fiber 3g
sugars 4g—with artificial
   sweetener 2g
protein 23g

Try this for a different tuna salad. The taste of curry and the crunch of water chestnuts make this especially good.

Makes 3 cups
4 servings

Each Serving
3/4 cup

Carb Servings
1/2

Exchanges
1 vegetable
3 lean meat

Nutrient Analysis
calories 165
total fat 6g
saturated fat 1g
cholesterol 36mg
sodium 484mg
total carbohydrate 7g
dietary fiber 1g
sugars 1g
protein 20g

Curry Tuna Salad

1 teaspoon dried or 1 tablespoon fresh minced onion
1 tablespoon lemon juice
2 cans (6 ounces each) water pack tuna, drained
1 can (8 ounces) sliced water chestnuts, drained
1/4 cup light mayonnaise
2 teaspoons lite soy sauce
1 teaspoon curry powder
lettuce leaves

Mix onion with lemon juice and let set for 5 minutes.

Combine tuna and water chestnuts in a small bowl.

Make dressing by mixing mayonnaise, onion, lemon juice, soy sauce, and curry. Combine dressing with tuna and water chestnuts. Serve on a bed of lettuce.

VARIATION: *Toasted Tuna Sandwich*–Spread 1/2 cup of tuna salad on half of a toasted whole-grain English muffin. Heat under broiler until hot.

Shrimp Coleslaw

1 small head of cabbage, shredded (about 5 cups)
1 medium green pepper, diced
1 carrot, chopped
2 green onions, chopped
2 cups cooked and cleaned shrimp

Dressing:

1 cup fat-free plain yogurt
3 tablespoons rice vinegar
1 tablespoon sugar or the equivalent in artificial
   sweetener
2 teaspoons dried dill weed
1/2 teaspoon ground black pepper
1/2 teaspoon celery seed
1/2 teaspoon Dijon mustard

In a large bowl, combine vegetables with shrimp.

Mix dressing ingredients and pour over
vegetables. Serve immediately or chill
for 1 hour before serving.

*Try this colorful coleslaw.
It's low in fat because
fat-free yogurt is used for
part of the dressing. Fresh
or imitation crab can be
substituted for the shrimp.*

Makes 8 cups
8 servings

Each Serving
1 cup

Carb Servings
1/2

Exchanges
2 vegetable
1 lean meat

Nutrient Analysis
calories 86—with artificial
   sweetener 80
total fat 1g
saturated fat 0g
cholesterol 76mg
sodium 140mg
total carbohydrate 10g—
   with artificial sweetener
   8g
dietary fiber 2g
sugars 7g—with artificial
   sweetener 5g
protein 11g

This is a great main-dish salad for a warm day. Serve with a whole-grain roll to complete the meal.

Makes 12 cups
5 servings

Each Serving
2 1/2 cups

Carb Servings
1—with artificial
  sweetener 1/2

Exchanges
1/2 carbohydrate
1 vegetable—0 with
  artificial sweetener
3 lean meat
1 1/2 fat

Nutrient Analysis
calories 247—with
  artificial sweetener 228
total fat 12g
saturated fat 2g
cholesterol 175mg
sodium 230mg
total carbohydrate 14g—
  with artificial sweetener
  9g
dietary fiber 5g
sugars 7g—with artificial
  sweetener 2g
protein 24g

Shrimp Salad

2 tablespoons sugar or the equivalent in artificial
  sweetener
3/4 cup rice vinegar
1 medium avocado, peeled and sliced
1/2 cup chopped green onion
1/4 cup chopped fresh cilantro
1/4 teaspoon crushed red pepper
1/4 teaspoon garlic powder
10–12 ounces salad greens (about 2 quarts)
1 pound cooked and cleaned salad shrimp
1/2 cup coarsely chopped dry-roasted, unsalted peanuts

In a medium bowl, mix sugar with rice vinegar and stir to dissolve.

Add the next five ingredients and mix well.

Just before serving, mix salad greens with the shrimp and dressing in a large serving bowl. Top with peanuts.

NOTE: One serving is an excellent source of fiber.

Most of the fat in this recipe is heart-healthy monounsaturated fat.

Seafood Salad

1 pound imitation or fresh crab
1 cup chopped celery
1/4 cup chopped green onion
2 tablespoons light mayonnaise
2 tablespoons fat-free plain yogurt
1 tablespoon lemon juice
1/4 teaspoon paprika
1/4 cup (1 ounce) grated, reduced-fat cheddar cheese

Combine the first three ingredients in a medium bowl.

In a small bowl, combine mayonnaise, yogurt, lemon juice, and paprika. Stir in cheese. Add to crab and mix well.

VARIATION: *Toasted Seafood Salad Sandwich*–Spread 1/2 cup on a toasted whole-grain English muffin half and broil until cheese is melted.

This recipe is good on lettuce or as a sandwich spread. Substituting shrimp for part, or all, of the crab also tastes good. Sodium can be reduced by using fresh crab instead of the imitation.

Makes 4 cups
8 servings

Each Serving
1/2 cup

Carb Servings
1/2

Exchanges
1 vegetable
1 lean meat

Nutrient Analysis
calories 85
total fat 3g
saturated fat 1g
cholesterol 15mg
sodium 544mg
total carbohydrate 7g
dietary fiber 0g
sugars 1g
protein 8g

Rice, Beans, and Potatoes

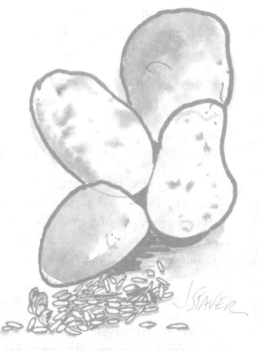

Brown rice, potatoes with the skin, and beans all add fiber to your diet. Using quick-cooking brown rice reduces cooking time by as much as 30 minutes.

This is a colorful side dish that you can vary by using different root vegetables such as parsnips, turnips, and sweet potatoes.

Makes 4 cups
4 servings

Each Serving
1 cup

Carb Servings
1 1/2

Exchanges
1 starch
1 vegetable
1/2 fat

Nutrient Analysis
calories 131
total fat 4g
saturated fat 1g
cholesterol 0mg
sodium 51mg
total carbohydrate 23g
dietary fiber 4g
sugars 5g
protein 2g

Roasted Root Vegetables

4 small thin-skinned new potatoes, not peeled (about 3/4 pound)
2 cups whole baby carrots
1 onion, cut in eighths
1 tablespoon chopped garlic
1 tablespoon olive oil
1/4 teaspoon dried thyme
1/4 teaspoon dried rosemary
1/4 teaspoon ground black pepper
1/4 teaspoon salt (optional)

Preheat to 475 degrees.

Cut each potato into eight wedges. Add to a large bowl along with the carrots and onions. Add remaining ingredients and toss to coat.

Arrange vegetables, so that they are not crowded, in a 9-inch by 13-inch baking pan that has been sprayed with nonstick cooking spray. Roast 15 minutes. Stir and turn vegetables. Return to oven for an additional 15 minutes or until vegetables are tender.

NOTE: One serving is a good source of fiber.

COOKING TIP: Oven temperature can be lowered so these can bake alongside another dish. Lowering the temperature will increase the cooking time.

Cheese-Stuffed Potatoes

4 medium baked potatoes, about 5 ounces each
    (still warm)
1 cup low-fat cottage cheese or low-fat Ricotta cheese
1 tablespoon fat-free milk
2 tablespoons chopped green onion
1/4 teaspoon paprika

Slice each potato in half, lengthwise. Scoop out pulp,
leaving about 1/4-inch thick shells.

Blend cheese, milk, and potato pulp. Mash until smooth.
Add onion. Fill potato shell halves with mixture.

Arrange potatoes on a baking dish and sprinkle with
paprika. Use a microwave-safe dish if cooking in
microwave.

Follow directions below for microwave or conventional
oven.

MICROWAVE OVEN: Cover with wax paper. Heat on high
for 5 minutes, turning 1/4 turn halfway through cooking.

CONVENTIONAL OVEN: Preheat oven to 350 degrees.
Bake for 10–15 minutes or until thoroughly heated.

*This is a potato dish that
kids like. The addition
of cheese adds a good
flavor. For a creamier
texture, process cottage
cheese and milk in a
blender or food processor
until smooth before
mashing with potato.*

Makes 8 servings

Each Serving
1 potato half

Carb Servings
1

Exchanges
1 starch

Nutrient Analysis
calories 71
total fat 0g
saturated fat 0g
cholesterol 1mg
sodium 120mg
total carbohydrate 12g
dietary fiber 2g
sugars 2g
protein 5g

This is easy to assemble and quick cooking if you're using a microwave. However, if you're not in a hurry, you'll find it is just as easy to use the oven. See the variation below for making this a main dish.

Makes 6 servings

Each Serving

Carb Servings
1 1/2

Exchanges
1 1/2 starch

Nutrient Analysis
calories 107
total fat 0g
saturated fat 0g
cholesterol 1mg
sodium 62mg
total carbohydrate 22g
dietary fiber 3g
sugars 5g
protein 4g

Scalloped Potatoes

6–8 new potatoes, not peeled (about 4 cups, sliced)
2 tablespoons unbleached all-purpose flour
1 tablespoon dried or 1/4 cup fresh minced onion
1 teaspoon fat-free butter-flavored sprinkles
1/4 teaspoon ground black pepper
1 1/2 cups fat-free milk

Spray a 2 1/2-quart casserole dish with nonstick cooking spray. Use a microwave-safe dish if cooking in the microwave.

Cut potatoes into 1/4-inch slices. Layer potatoes in the casserole, sprinkling each layer with flour, onion, butter sprinkles, and pepper. Pour milk over top. Follow directions below for microwave or conventional oven.

MICROWAVE OVEN: Cook, covered, 15–18 minutes, stirring every 4 minutes. Be sure to use a container twice the size of the contents to prevent a boil-over.

CONVENTIONAL OVEN: Preheat oven to 350 degrees. Bake uncovered about 1 1/4 hours. Stir two to three times during cooking.

NOTE: One serving is a good source of fiber.

VARIATION: *Scalloped Potatoes with Meat*–To make this a main dish, add cubed ham or smoked turkey sausage before cooking. Top with 2 ounces grated, reduced-fat cheese.

Low-Fat French Fries

4 medium potatoes, not peeled (about 5 ounces each)
1 tablespoon oil (canola or olive)
salt to taste (optional)
malt vinegar to taste (optional)

Preheat oven to 475 degrees.

Cut potatoes into half-inch slices or strips. Place potato slices in a plastic bag with oil and shake well to coat potatoes evenly.

Spray a baking sheet with nonstick cooking spray. Arrange potatoes in a single layer and bake for 30 minutes, or until golden brown, turning potatoes every 10 minutes.

Sprinkle with salt (optional), and serve with malt vinegar (optional).

NOTE: One serving is a good source of fiber.

VARIATION: Temperature can be decreased to 450 degrees and baking time increased to 40 minutes.

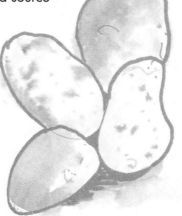

This is a favorite for children and adults that is so easy to prepare! The best part is these fries are low in fat.

Makes 4 servings

Each Serving

Carb Servings
1 1/2

Exchanges
1 1/2 starch
1/2 fat

Nutrient Analysis
calories 129
total fat 4g
saturated fat 0g
cholesterol 0mg
sodium 8mg
total carbohydrate 22g
dietary fiber 3g
sugars 2g
protein 2g

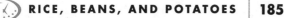

You can use either yams or sweet potatoes. The yams have a bright orange color and a stronger flavor. The sweet potatoes have a white color and a milder flavor. We prefer the taste of the sweet potatoes.

Makes 4 servings

Each Serving

Carb Servings
1

Exchanges
1 starch
1/2 fat

Nutrient Analysis
calories 116
total fat 4g
saturated fat 0g
cholesterol 0mg
sodium 15mg
total carbohydrate 20g
dietary fiber 3g
sugars 4g
protein 2g

Sweet Potato Fries

4 medium sweet potatoes or yams, peeled
(about 4 ounces each)
1 tablespoon oil (canola or olive)
salt to taste (optional)

Preheat oven to 450 degrees.

Cut potatoes into half-inch slices or strips. Place potato slices in a plastic bag with oil and shake well to coat potatoes evenly.

Spray a baking sheet with nonstick cooking spray. Arrange potatoes in a single layer and bake for 12–15 minutes, or until golden brown, turning potatoes halfway through cooking.

Sprinkle with salt (optional).

NOTE: One serving is a good source of fiber.

Herb Rice Blend

1 1/2 cups fat-free beef or chicken broth*
1 teaspoon dried or 1 tablespoon fresh minced onion
1/4 teaspoon dried marjoram
1/4 teaspoon dried thyme
1/8 teaspoon dried rosemary
1 1/2 cups uncooked quick-cooking brown rice

Mix the first five ingredients in a saucepan. Bring to a boil. Add rice and reduce heat to low. Cover and simmer for
5 minutes. Remove from heat and let stand 5 minutes before serving.

VARIATION: *Italian Herb Rice Blend*—Substitute 3/4 teaspoon Italian seasoning for the rosemary, marjoram, and thyme.

Sodium is figured for reduced sodium.

Quick-cooking brown rice makes this a quick dish. The addition of herbs adds a great flavor without additional calories.

Makes 2 cups
4 servings

Each Serving
1/2 cup

Carb Servings
2

Exchanges
2 starch

Nutrient Analysis
calories 136
total fat 1g
saturated fat 0g
cholesterol 0mg
sodium 150mg
total carbohydrate 26g
dietary fiber 2g
sugars 0g
protein 4g

You can vary the vegetables if you want more color or crunch. This is a good way to change a plain rice dish and you can even use leftover vegetables.

Makes 3 cups
4 servings

Each Serving
3/4 cup

Carb Servings
2

Exchanges
2 starch

Nutrient Analysis
calories 142
total fat 1g
saturated fat 0g
cholesterol 0mg
sodium 151mg
total carbohydrate 27g
dietary fiber 2g
sugars 1g
protein 5g

Herb and Vegetable Rice Blend

1 recipe Herb Rice Blend (page 187)
1 cup cooked, sliced vegetables (such as mushrooms, celery, etc.)

Prepare one full recipe of Herb Rice Blend.

Add hot vegetables and mix well.

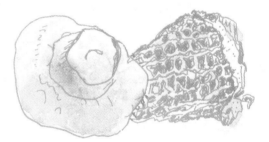

 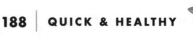

Ranch Beans

1 can (16 ounces) fat-free baked beans
1 can (15 ounces) red kidney beans, drained and rinsed
1/2 cup chopped green pepper
2 tablespoons catsup
2 tablespoons molasses
1 tablespoon Dijon mustard
1/2 teaspoon dried or 2 teaspoons fresh minced onion

STOVETOP: Place all ingredients in saucepan and heat thoroughly (about 10 minutes).

MICROWAVE OVEN: Place all ingredients in a microwave-safe bowl. Cover and cook on high for 5 minutes, stirring halfway through cooking time.

NOTE: One serving is an excellent source of fiber.

Try this "dressed up" version of baked beans. It can be served as a side dish or as a main dish.

Makes 3 cups
6 servings

Each Serving
1/2 cup

Carb Servings
2

Exchanges
2 starch

Nutrient Analysis
calories 160
total fat 0g
saturated fat 0g
cholesterol 0mg
sodium 472mg
total carbohydrate 31g
dietary fiber 9g
sugars 8g
protein 8g

Sandwiches and Pizza

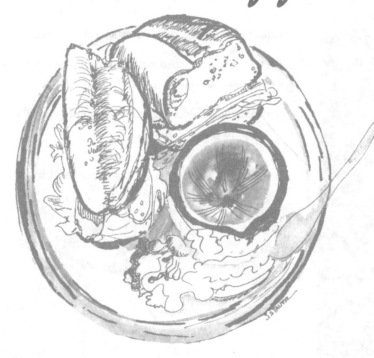

Try these recipes for lunch or a quick supper. Use whole-grain breads to increase the fiber in your diet.

Leftover turkey or sliced turkey from the deli is good in this sandwich. You can omit the cheese and use just turkey. If you're in a hurry, heat the sandwiches in the microwave.

Makes 4 sandwiches

Each Serving
1 sandwich

Carb Servings
2

Exchanges
2 starch
3 lean meat

Nutrient Analysis
calories 273
total fat 5g
saturated fat 2g
cholesterol 56mg
sodium 424mg
total carbohydrate 31g
dietary fiber 4g
sugars 5g
protein 26g

Turkey French Dips

8 ounces cooked turkey slices
4 long whole-grain rolls, 2 ounces each
2 ounces grated (1/2 cup) reduced-fat mozzarella cheese
1 package au jus gravy mix

Preheat oven to 400 degrees.

Cut rolls lengthwise. Place two ounces of turkey and one-fourth of the mozzarella cheese on each roll. Wrap each roll in aluminum foil and heat in the oven for 10 minutes.

Prepare au jus according to package directions or add more water to reduce the sodium content.

Slice each sandwich in half, diagonally. Serve each with 1/3 cup au jus.

NOTE: One serving is a good source of fiber.

Tomato and Ricotta Sandwich

1 slice whole-grain toast
1/4 cup low-fat Ricotta cheese
2 tomato slices
1/2 teaspoon Dijon mustard

Preheat broiler.

Spread cheese on toast. Top with tomato. Spread mustard on tomato. Broil until tomato is hot.

NOTE: One serving is a good source of fiber.

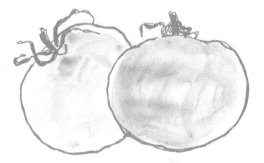

Serve this for a quick lunch. The addition of mustard adds a good flavor.

Makes 1 sandwich

Each Serving

Carb Servings
1

Exchanges
1 starch
1 vegetable
1 lean meat

Nutrient Analysis
calories 138
total fat 3g
saturated fat 1g
cholesterol 15mg
sodium 283mg
total carbohydrate 20g
dietary fiber 4g
sugars 12g
protein 10g

This is especially quick to put together if you remember to thaw the bread dough overnight. Change the filling ingredients to suit your taste.

Crusty Calzone

Crust:
1 pound frozen whole-wheat bread dough, thawed and at room temperature*
1/4 cup pizza sauce
1/2 teaspoon garlic powder
1/4 teaspoon Italian seasoning

Turkey Sausage Filling:
1/2 pound low-fat turkey smoked sausage, sliced very thin
1 green pepper, sliced
1/2 onion, sliced thin
1 cup (4 ounces) grated, reduced-fat cheese

Ground Meat Filling:
1/2 pound extra lean ground beef or ground turkey (7% fat, cooked and crumbled)
1 cup thinly sliced vegetables
1 cup (4 ounces) grated, reduced-fat cheese (mozzarella or cheddar)

Preheat oven to 425 degrees. Roll dough into 10-inch by 14-inch rectangle. Place on a baking sheet that has been sprayed with nonstick cooking spray.

Spread pizza sauce on half of the dough. Sprinkle with garlic powder and Italian seasoning. Top with filling ingredients.

Fold dough over and press edges together to seal in filling. Bake for 20 minutes. Cut into eight slices.

NOTE: One serving is a good source of fiber.

The recipe using the sausage filling is higher in sodium and should be limited by those on a low-sodium diet.

Thaw frozen bread dough in refrigerator overnight, then set out for about 1/2 hour at room temperature for easier rolling.

Makes 8 servings

Each Serving
1 slice

Carb Servings
2

Exchanges
2 starch
2 lean meat

Nutrient Analysis (Sausage Filling)
calories 237
total fat 7g
saturated fat 2g
cholesterol 25mg
sodium 684mg
total carbohydrate 30g
dietary fiber 3g
sugars 4g
protein 15g

Nutrient Analysis (Ground Meat Filling)
calories 230
total fat 6g
saturated fat 2g
cholesterol 25mg
sodium 435mg
total carbohydrate 29g
dietary fiber 3g
sugars 3g
protein 17g

These are a family favorite for a quick supper. Just add a tossed salad. I use meatballs that I have frozen, so it really is quick.

Makes 4 sandwiches

Each Serving
1 sandwich

Carb Servings
2 1/2

Exchanges
2 starch
1 vegetable
2 lean meat

Nutrient Analysis
calories 331
total fat 10g
saturated fat 3g
cholesterol 47mg
sodium 610mg
total carbohydrate 40g
dietary fiber 6g
sugars 9g
protein 23g

Meatball Sandwich

16 Baked Meatballs (page 291)
1 cup spaghetti sauce (less than 4 g fat per 4 ounces)
4 long whole-grain rolls, 2 ounces each

Heat meatballs in spaghetti sauce.

Slice rolls lengthwise, being careful not to cut through the last half inch of the roll. Fill each roll with 4 meatballs and 1/4 of the sauce.

NOTE: One serving is an excellent source of fiber.

Individual Pizza

2 whole-grain English muffins
1/2 cup pizza sauce
4 ounces cooked turkey slices
1/2 cup (2 ounces) grated, reduced-fat mozzarella cheese
1/4 cup thinly sliced green pepper
1/4 cup thinly sliced onion

Preheat oven to 475 degrees.

Cut muffins in half and spread pizza sauce over each half. Top with turkey, cheese, and vegetables.

Bake for 15 minutes or until cheese is melted.

NOTE: One serving is a good source of fiber.

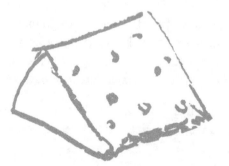

This is a quick pizza recipe. Try this one for lunch or as a quick after-school snack.

Makes 4 pizzas

Each Serving
1 pizza

Carb Servings
1

Exchanges
1 starch
2 lean meat

Nutrient Analysis
calories 159
total fat 3g
saturated fat 1g
cholesterol 31mg
sodium 421mg
total carbohydrate 16g
dietary fiber 3g
sugars 5g
protein 16g

This pizza is piled high with vegetables that have been roasted with Italian seasonings. You'll use about 8 cups of vegetables and you can vary the vegetables to your liking.

Makes 12 slices
6 servings

Each Serving
2 slices

Carb Servings
2

Exchanges
1 1/2 starch
2 vegetable
1 medium-fat meat

Nutrient Analysis
calories 238
total fat 6g
saturated fat 2g
cholesterol 10mg
sodium 455mg
total carbohydrate 34g
dietary fiber 5g
sugars 6g
protein 12g

Piled-High Vegetable Pizza

1 small eggplant, not peeled (about 12–14 ounces), cut into one-inch cubes (about 4 cups)
1 onion, chopped
1 cup chopped bell pepper, green or yellow
1 tablespoon chopped garlic
1 teaspoon Italian seasoning
1/2 teaspoon salt (optional)
1/4 teaspoon ground black pepper
2 medium tomatoes, chopped (about 2 cups)
1 (10-ounce) thin pizza crust (such as Boboli)
1/2 cup pizza sauce
1 cup (4 ounces) grated reduced-fat mozzarella cheese
1/4 cup Parmesan cheese (optional)

Preheat oven to 450 degrees.

In a large bowl, mix vegetables, except tomatoes, with garlic and seasonings. Spread in a 9-inch by 13-inch baking pan that has been sprayed with nonstick cooking spray. Roast for 12–15 minutes. Add tomatoes and return to oven for 5 minutes or until all vegetables are tender. Drain any liquid.

While vegetables are roasting, place pizza crust on a baking pan. Spread pizza sauce over crust and top with cheese.

Bake for 8–10 minutes alongside the vegetables. Top with roasted vegetables and Parmesan cheese. Cut into 12 slices.

NOTE: One serving is an excellent source of fiber.

Boboli Pizza
Shrimp Style

1 (10-ounce) thin pizza crust (such as Boboli)
1/2 cup seafood cocktail sauce
1 cup (4 ounces) grated, reduced-fat cheese (mozzarella
  or cheddar)
2 cups cooked and cleaned shrimp

Preheat oven to 450 degrees. Place pizza crust on pizza pan. Spread cocktail sauce on the pizza crust. Top with cheese. Bake for 5 minutes.

Top with shrimp and continue to cook for 3–5 minutes or just until shrimp is heated and cheese is melted.

NOTE: This recipe is higher in sodium and should be limited by those on a low-sodium diet.

Seafood cocktail sauce adds a different taste to a traditional food. This would also be good served as an appetizer.

Makes 12 slices
6 servings

Each Serving
2 slices

Carb Servings
2

Exchanges
1 1/2 starch
1 vegetable
2 lean meat

Nutrient Analysis
calories 259
total fat 6g
saturated fat 2g
cholesterol 110mg
sodium 708mg
total carbohydrate 28g
dietary fiber 1g
sugars 5g
protein 21g

Complete this meal by adding fresh fruit or a tossed salad. See the variation below for reducing calories and carbohydrate.

Makes 5 sandwiches

Each Serving
1 sandwich (1/2 cup filling)

Carb Servings
2 1/2

Exchanges
2 starch
2 vegetable
3 lean meat

Nutrient Analysis
calories 336
total fat 10g
saturated fat 3g
cholesterol 56mg
sodium 594mg
total carbohydrate 40g
dietary fiber 5g
sugars 11g
protein 24g

Sloppy Joes

1 pound extra-lean ground beef or ground turkey (7% fat)
3/4 cup chopped onion
1 tablespoon chopped garlic
1 can (10.75 ounces) condensed tomato soup*
2 teaspoons prepared mustard
5 whole-grain hamburger buns (2 ounces each)

MICROWAVE OVEN: In a microwave-safe bowl, crumble meat and add onion and garlic. Cook on high for 4 minutes, turning halfway through cooking time. Add soup and mustard. Continue cooking for about 2 minutes or until heated thoroughly.

STOVETOP: Brown meat with onion and garlic in a skillet that has been sprayed with nonstick cooking spray. Add soup and mustard. Simmer for about 10 minutes.

Spoon meat mixture on 5 bun halves. Top with remaining buns. For a crisp texture, place filled buns on a baking sheet and bake at 475 degrees for 5–10 minutes before serving.

NOTE: One serving is an excellent source of fiber.

VARIATION: *Open-Faced Sloppy Joes*–Spoon 1/2 cup meat mixture on half a bun and serve open-face. One serving is 260 calories and 25 grams of carbohydrate.

*Sodium is figured for reduced sodium.

Meatless Entrees

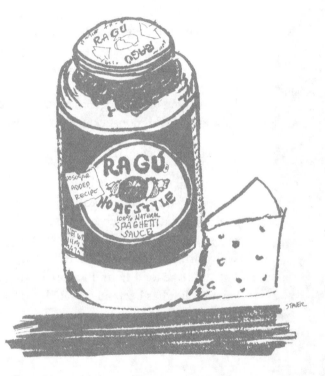

Use low-fat cheeses to cut back on fat and reduce calories. Sharp cheese is a good choice, as it has a stronger flavor. Use egg substitute when limiting whole eggs. Add lots of vegetables to your meals, as they add fiber and color to your diet.

You don't precook the noodles in this recipe, so it is really fast to assemble. This can be put together the night before and refrigerated without baking.

Makes 12 servings

Each Serving

Carb Servings
2

Exchanges
1 1/2 starch
1 vegetable
1 lean meat

Nutrient Analysis
calories 218
total fat 5g
saturated fat 2g
cholesterol 9mg
sodium 596mg
total carbohydrate 28g
dietary fiber 2g
sugars 6g
protein 15g

Quick Lasagna

3 cups low-fat cottage cheese or low-fat Ricotta cheese
2 tablespoons dried parsley
1 teaspoon chopped garlic
4 cups spaghetti sauce (less than 4 grams fat per 4 ounces)*
3/4 pound uncooked lasagna noodles (12 noodles)
1 cup (4 ounces) grated, reduced-fat mozzarella cheese
1/4 cup grated Parmesan cheese

Preheat oven to 350 degrees. Spray a 9-inch by 13-inch baking pan with nonstick cooking spray.

Mix cottage cheese, parsley, and garlic.

Pour 1 cup of sauce in bottom of pan. Layer in this order: 4 noodles, 1/2 cheese mixture, 1/2 mozzarella, 1 cup sauce, 4 noodles, 1/2 cheese mixture, 1/2 mozzarella, 1 cup sauce, 4 noodles, and the rest of the sauce. Sprinkle with Parmesan cheese. Covered tightly with aluminum foil and bake for 1 hour. Increase baking time by 15 minutes if it has been refrigerated.

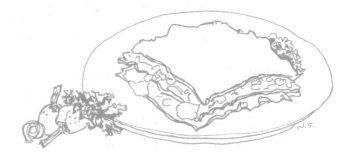

Or one jar (1 pound, 10 ounces) and water to equal 4 cups.

 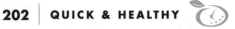

Tomato and Basil Pasta

4 medium tomatoes, diced (4 cups)
2 teaspoons dried basil
2 teaspoons chopped garlic
1 teaspoon salt (optional)
1/4 teaspoon ground black pepper
6 ounces uncooked angel hair pasta
grated Parmesan cheese (optional)

Mix the first five ingredients and let set at room temperature at least 1 hour.

Cook angel hair pasta according to package directions and drain.

Top pasta with tomato mixture. Serve immediately and top with Parmesan cheese (optional).

NOTE: One serving is a good source of fiber.

Fresh tomatoes and basil add a wonderful flavor to this light dish.

Makes 6 cups
4 servings

Each Serving
1 1/2 cups

Carb Servings
2 1/2

Exchanges
2 starch
2 vegetable

Nutrient Analysis
calories 193
total fat 1g
saturated fat 0g
cholesterol 0mg
sodium 9mg
total carbohydrate 39g
dietary fiber 4g
sugars 6g
protein 8g

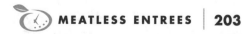

This has a great flavor. Try adding shrimp for variety.

Makes 4 servings

Each Serving

Carb Servings
1 1/2

Exchanges
1 starch
1 vegetable

Nutrient Analysis
calories 109
total fat 1g
saturated fat 0g
cholesterol 1mg
sodium 41mg
total carbohydrate 22g
dietary fiber 3g
sugars 6g
protein 5g

Italian Broccoli and Pasta

2 cups uncooked fettuccini noodles (eggless)
2 cups broccoli florets
3 tablespoons chopped green onion
1 can (14.5 ounces) diced tomatoes*, not drained
1/2 teaspoon dried thyme
1/2 teaspoon dried oregano
1/2 teaspoon ground black pepper
2 teaspoons grated Parmesan cheese

Cook fettuccini according to package directions and drain.

Spray a skillet with nonstick cooking spray. Add broccoli and onion and stir-fry for 3 minutes. Add tomatoes and seasonings and simmer until heated throughout.

Spoon vegetable mixture over fettuccini and top with Parmesan cheese.

NOTE: One serving is a good source of fiber.

Sodium is figured for no added salt.

Vegetables Primavera

4 cups vegetables, any combination of the following:
   chopped: broccoli, cauliflower, celery, cabbage,
            eggplant, onions
   sliced: mushrooms, green peppers, carrots
   whole: pea pods, green beans
1 jar (26 ounces) spaghetti sauce (less than 4 grams
   fat per 4 ounces)
2 1/2 cups cooked spaghetti noodles (3 ounces dry)

MICROWAVE OVEN: Mix vegetables and spaghetti sauce
in a microwave-safe dish. Cover and cook on high for 15
minutes, stirring at 5-minute intervals. Cook longer if you
prefer vegetables to be less crisp.

STOVETOP: Mix vegetables and spaghetti sauce in a
saucepan. Cover and simmer until vegetables are cooked
to preferred tenderness.

Serve cooked vegetables and sauce over noodles.

NOTE: One serving is an excellent
        source of fiber.

*Children may not like
all the vegetables in this
recipe, but adults sure
do. Top with Parmesan
cheese when serving.*

Makes 5 servings

Each Serving

Carb Servings
2

Exchanges
1 starch
3 vegetable

Nutrient Analysis
calories 169
total fat 3g
saturated fat 1g
cholesterol 0mg
sodium 616mg
total carbohydrate 29g
dietary fiber 5g
sugars 11g
protein 6g

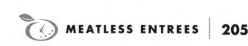

This is a good way to use zucchini, and it is a delicious supper or breakfast dish.

Makes 4 servings

Each Serving

Carb Servings
1/2

Exchanges
1 vegetable
1 lean meat

Nutrient Analysis
calories 65
total fat 1g
saturated fat 0g
cholesterol 2mg
sodium 168mg
total carbohydrate 6g
dietary fiber 1g
sugars 3g
protein 9g

Italian Zucchini Frittata

4 cups unpeeled, grated zucchini (about 1 1/2 pounds)
2 tablespoons chopped onion
1/2 teaspoon chopped garlic
1 cup egg substitute (equal to 4 eggs)
2 tablespoons fat-free milk
1/2 teaspoon dried oregano
1/2 teaspoon dried basil
1/2 teaspoon salt (optional)
1/4 teaspoon ground black pepper
2 tablespoons grated Parmesan cheese

Preheat broiler. Spray a 10-inch skillet with nonstick cooking spray.

Sauté the first three ingredients until zucchini is tender, pouring off any liquid.

Meanwhile, mix eggs, milk, and seasonings. Add to the zucchini mixture and cook until the eggs begin to set.

Top with Parmesan cheese. Broil just until top is golden.

Spanish Zucchini Frittata

4 cups unpeeled, grated zucchini (about 1 1/2 pounds)
2 tablespoons chopped onion
1/2 teaspoon chopped garlic
1 can (4 ounces) diced green chiles
1 cup egg substitute (equal to 4 eggs)
2 tablespoons fat-free milk
1/2 teaspoon ground cumin
1/2 teaspoon chili powder
1/2 teaspoon salt (optional)
1/4 teaspoon ground black pepper
salsa (optional)

Preheat broiler. Spray a 10-inch skillet with nonstick cooking spray.

Sauté the first three ingredients until zucchini is tender, pouring off any liquid. Add chiles.

Meanwhile, mix eggs, milk, and seasonings. Add to the zucchini mixture and cook until the eggs begin to set.

Broil just until top is golden. Serve with salsa.

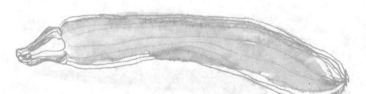

This is one of my favorite omelets. I like the combination of chiles, salsa, and eggs.

Makes 4 servings

Each Serving

Carb Servings
1/2

Exchanges
1 vegetable
1 lean meat

Nutrient Analysis
calories 59
total fat 0g
saturated fat 0g
cholesterol 0mg
sodium 221mg
total carbohydrate 7g
dietary fiber 2g
sugars 3g
protein 8g

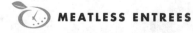

Poultry

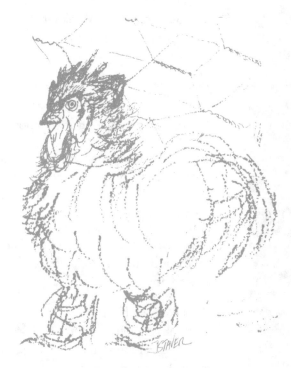

Poultry is a lean choice if the skin and fat are removed. Keep some skinless, boneless pieces in the freezer for last-minute meals.

This Asian dish has a unique flavor. The optional toppings of mint, green onion, and peanuts allow you to individualize your wrap. Serve as an hors d'oeuvre, as a main dish, or stuffed in pita bread halves.

Makes 12 wraps
4 servings

Each Serving
3 wraps

Carb Servings
0

Exchanges
3 lean meat

Nutrient Analysis
calories 131
total fat 2g
saturated fat 0g
cholesterol 65mg
sodium 77mg
total carbohydrate 2g
dietary fiber 1g
sugars 0g
protein 26g

Chicken Lettuce Wraps

1 pound skinless, boneless chicken breasts, cut into bite-size pieces
2 tablespoons minced fresh ginger
1/2 teaspoon salt (optional)
1/4 teaspoon ground black pepper
1/2 cup chopped fresh cilantro
12 large lettuce leaves (bib or butter)

Optional Toppings:
green onion, sliced
mint leaves, chopped
dry-roasted peanuts, coarsely chopped

In a medium saucepan, that has been sprayed with nonstick cooking spray, sauté chicken with ginger for a few minutes, until chicken is no longer pink. Season with salt and pepper. Add cilantro.

To serve: Arrange a bowl of chicken mixture, lettuce leaves, and optional toppings on serving area.

To make each lettuce wrap, place about 1/4 cup of chicken mixture in a lettuce leaf. Add optional toppings. Roll up and enjoy!

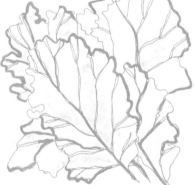

Cooked and Cubed Chicken

1 3/4 pounds skinless, boneless chicken breasts

Follow directions below for microwave or conventional oven.

MICROWAVE OVEN: Cut breasts into 1-inch strips. Arrange on a microwave-safe baking dish in a circle on the outer portion of the dish. Cover with wax paper and microwave on high for 5 minutes, rearranging halfway through cooking time. Let set a few minutes before cutting into bite-size pieces.

STOVETOP METHOD: Place chicken in a saucepan and cover with water. Cover and simmer on low until tender (about 15–20 minutes). Drain liquid and save for making soup. Cut into bite-size pieces.

Cooked and cubed chicken is used in the following recipes:
Baked Chimichangas
Cabbage and Chicken Salad
Chicken and Fruit Salad
Chicken and Spinach Salad
Chicken Enchiladas
Chicken in a Pocket
Chicken Tortilla Casserole
Chinese Chicken Salad
Cinnamon Chicken Salad
Green Chile Chicken Enchilada Casserole
Oriental Rice and Chicken Salad

Many recipes call for cooked chicken. You can use leftover turkey or leftover chicken, but when leftovers are not available, it's easy to microwave or simmer chicken. Cook extra and freeze for future use.

Makes 4 cups
8 servings

Each Serving
1/2 cup

Carb Servings
0

Exchanges
3 lean meat

Nutrient Analysis
calories 108
total fat 1g
saturated fat 0g
cholesterol 57mg
sodium 64mg
total carbohydrate 0g
dietary fiber 0g
sugars 0g
protein 23g

This recipe will become a family favorite. This also tastes great as a cold leftover without the sauce. Look for biscuits that are only 100 calories, 1.5 grams of fat, and 1 gram of fiber for 2 biscuits.

Makes 5 pockets
5 servings

Each Serving
1 pocket plus sauce

Carb Servings
2

Exchanges
2 starch
3 lean meat

Nutrient Analysis
calories 249
total fat 4g
saturated fat 1g
cholesterol 46mg
sodium 785mg
total carbohydrate 26g
dietary fiber 2g
sugars 5g
protein 27g

Chicken in a Pocket

2 cups cooked chicken, chopped or shredded
1 package (8 ounces) fat-free cream cheese (room temperature)
4 green onions, chopped
1 can (7 ounces) buttermilk biscuits (10 biscuits per can)

Sauce:
1/2 can (5 ounces) low-fat, condensed cream of chicken soup*
1/2 cup water

Preheat oven to 375 degrees. Mix the first three ingredients in a medium bowl.

Lay out half the biscuits on a baking sheet that has been sprayed with nonstick cooking spray. Lightly flatten the biscuits with the palm of your hand. Spoon part of the chicken mixture on five biscuits, reserving some filling for the sauce. Flatten remaining biscuits and place over biscuits topped with filling. Seal edges by pinching. Bake for 20 minutes or until biscuits are golden brown.

Meanwhile, prepare sauce by mixing the soup, water, and reserved filling. Heat in a saucepan on the stove until thoroughly heated or cook in the microwave for 2 1/2 minutes on high, stirring halfway through cooking time. Serve over each pocket.

Sodium is figured for reduced sodium.

NOTE: This recipe is higher in sodium and should be limited by those on a low-sodium diet.

 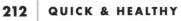

Polynesian Chicken

1 pound skinless, boneless chicken breasts or 2 pounds chicken parts, with bone
1/4 cup fat-free chicken broth*, or white wine
2 tablespoons lite soy sauce
2 tablespoons water
1 teaspoon hickory liquid smoke**
1/2 teaspoon ground ginger
1/4 cup brown sugar or the equivalent in artificial sweetener
1 teaspoon ground mustard

Skin chicken if parts are used. Mix the next five ingredients. Add chicken and marinate in the refrigerator for 1–3 hours.

Preheat oven to 350 degrees.

Add chicken and the marinade to a baking pan that has been sprayed with nonstick cooking spray. Be sure the pan is large enough so chicken pieces are not touching. Top chicken pieces with brown sugar and mustard. Bake for 30–40 minutes, or until chicken is no longer pink, basting during the last 15 minutes of cooking time. Serve with the sauce.

*Sodium is figured for reduced sodium.

**Hickory liquid smoke can be found in the grocery store next to the barbecue sauce.

The liquid smoke gives this dish an excellent flavor. The marinade becomes a delicious sauce that is especially good served over rice or noodles.

Makes 4 servings

Each Serving

Carb Servings
1—with artificial sweetener 0

Exchanges
1 carbohydrate—with artificial sweetener 0
3 lean meat

Nutrient Analysis
calories 186—with artificial sweetener 134
total fat 2g
saturated fat 0g
cholesterol 65mg
sodium 394mg
total carbohydrate 14g— with artificial sweetener 1g
dietary fiber 0g
sugars 13g—with artificial sweetener 0g
protein 27g

This recipe is a complete meal. It is very colorful and a good choice to serve when entertaining. Try tube-shaped or spiral pasta for variety.

Makes 9 cups
6 servings

Each Serving
1 1/2 cups

Carb Servings
1 1/2

Exchanges
1 1/2 starch
1 vegetable
2 lean meat

Nutrient Analysis
calories 213
total fat 2g
saturated fat 0g
cholesterol 43mg
sodium 89mg
total carbohydrate 25g
dietary fiber 3g
sugars 3g
protein 24g

Mediterranean Chicken

6 ounces pasta of your choice
1 pound skinless, boneless chicken breasts, cut into bite-size pieces
1 tablespoon chopped garlic
8 ounces sliced mushrooms (about 3 cups)
2 red bell peppers, chopped (about 2 cups)
2 cups broccoli florets, cut into bite-size pieces
1/2 teaspoon crushed red pepper
1/2 teaspoon Italian seasoning
1/4 teaspoon salt (optional)
1/8 teaspoon ground black pepper
1/2 cup fat-free chicken broth*
1 can (4 ounces) sliced black olives, drained (optional)
1/2 cup fat-free feta cheese (optional)

Cook pasta according to package directions. Drain.

Meanwhile, spray a large skillet with nonstick cooking spray. Add chicken to skillet and cook until chicken is no longer pink. Remove from skillet and keep warm.

Add vegetables and seasonings to skillet. Stir-fry for about 4–5 minutes until crisp-tender. Add water or broth, as needed, to prevent sticking. Add chicken, broth, and hot noodles to vegetables. Toss well. Cover and let set a couple of minutes before serving. If desired, top with feta cheese.

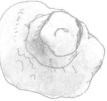

NOTE: One serving is a good source of fiber.

Sodium is figured for reduced sodium.

Chicken Breasts Florentine

2 tablespoons unbleached all-purpose flour
1/4 cup fat-free milk
3/4 cup fat-free chicken broth*
2 tablespoons grated Parmesan cheese
1/4 teaspoon salt (optional)
1/8 teaspoon ground black pepper
1/8 teaspoon ground nutmeg
2 packages (10 ounces each) frozen spinach, thawed, drained, and squeezed
1 1/2 pounds skinless, boneless, chicken breasts, cut into strips

Preheat oven to 375 degrees. Shake flour with milk in a covered container to prevent lumps. Mix flour mixture with chicken broth in a saucepan. Bring to a boil, stirring constantly, until thickened. Take off heat and stir in Parmesan cheese, salt, pepper, and nutmeg.

Mix spinach with 1/2 of the sauce and spread in a 9-inch by 13-inch baking pan that has been sprayed with nonstick cooking spray. Arrange chicken over spinach. Pour remainder of sauce over chicken. Sprinkle with additional nutmeg.

Bake, uncovered, for 20–25 minutes or until chicken is no longer pink.

Sodium is figured for reduced sodium.

This is a very simple and attractive dish. Fresh Parmesan cheese adds a good flavor to this recipe.

Makes 6 servings

Each Serving

Carb Servings
1/2

Exchanges
1 vegetable
3 lean meat

Nutrient Analysis
calories 164
total fat 2g
saturated fat 1g
cholesterol 67mg
sodium 205mg
total carbohydrate 6g
dietary fiber 2g
sugars 1g
protein 29g

This flavorful casserole has a delicious gravy. Serve as is or with brown rice or noodles.

Makes 5 servings

Each Serving

Carb Servings
1/2

Exchanges
2 vegetable
3 lean meat

Nutrient Analysis
calories 168
total fat 3g
saturated fat 1g
cholesterol 54mg
sodium 351mg
total carbohydrate 10g
dietary fiber 4g
sugars 2g
protein 25g

Chicken and Broccoli Casserole

1 pound skinless, boneless chicken breasts, cut into 8 strips
4 cups bite-size broccoli pieces
1 can (13 ounces) mushroom pieces and stems, drained and rinsed
1 can (10.75 ounces) low-fat, condensed cream of mushroom soup*
1/4 can water
1/2 teaspoon dried rosemary
1/4 teaspoon paprika
1/8 teaspoon ground black pepper

Preheat oven to 350 degrees. Arrange chicken in an 8-inch by 8-inch baking pan that has been sprayed with nonstick cooking spray. Top with vegetables.

Mix soup, water, and rosemary. Spread over chicken and vegetables. Sprinkle with paprika and pepper.

Bake, uncovered, for 50–60 minutes or until chicken is no longer pink and broccoli is tender. Let set 10 minutes before serving.

NOTE: One serving is a good source of fiber.

* *Sodium is figured for reduced sodium.*

Chicken and Vegetables in Gravy

1 1/2 pounds skinless, boneless chicken breasts or
  2 1/2–3 pounds chicken parts, skin removed

1 can (14 ounces) quartered artichoke hearts, drained
  and rinsed, or 2 cups of broccoli florets

1 can (13 ounces) mushroom pieces and stems, drained
  and rinsed

1/2 teaspoon paprika

1/4 teaspoon ground black pepper

1/3 cup unbleached all-purpose flour

1 1/2 cups fat-free chicken broth*, divided

1/3 cup dry sherry or chicken broth

1/2 teaspoon salt (optional)

1/2 teaspoon dried rosemary

Preheat oven to 350 degrees. If using chicken breasts, cut into strips.

Place chicken in a 9-inch by 13-inch baking pan that has been sprayed with nonstick cooking spray. Arrange artichoke hearts and mushrooms between chicken pieces. Sprinkle paprika and pepper over chicken.

In a covered container, shake flour with 1/2 cup of cold broth to prevent lumps. In a saucepan, add flour/broth mixture, remaining broth, dry sherry, salt, and rosemary. Heat on medium and bring to a boil, stirring constantly until thickened. Pour over chicken and bake for 40–50 minutes.

NOTE: One serving is a good source of fiber.

Sodium is figured for reduced sodium.

The artichokes give a tangy flavor or you can substitute broccoli. This makes a very good mushroom gravy.

Makes 6 servings

Each Serving

Carb Servings
1

Exchanges
1/2 starch
1 vegetable
3 lean meat

Nutrient Analysis
calories 192
total fat 2g
saturated fat 0g
cholesterol 65mg
sodium 337mg
total carbohydrate 11g
dietary fiber 4g
sugars 1g
protein 30g

This is a very easy one-dish meal. Look for biscuits that are only 100 calories, 1.5 grams of fat, and 1 gram of fiber for 2 biscuits. This recipe is good when using leftover turkey or chicken.

Makes 5 servings
5 cups plus 10 biscuits

Each Serving
1 cup and 2 biscuits

Carb Servings
2

Exchanges
1 1/2 starch
1 vegetable
3 lean meat

Nutrient Analysis
calories 261
total fat 3g
saturated fat 0g
cholesterol 52mg
sodium 586mg
total carbohydrate 31g
dietary fiber 3g
sugars 6g
protein 28g

Chicken and Biscuits

1/4 cup unbleached all-purpose flour
1 3/4 cups fat-free chicken broth*, divided
1 pound skinless, boneless chicken breasts, cut into cubes
1 cup frozen peas or corn
8 ounces sliced mushrooms (about 3 cups)
1 jar (2 ounces) chopped pimiento, drained
1 teaspoon dried parsley
1/8 teaspoon ground black pepper
1 can (7 ounces) buttermilk biscuits (10 biscuits per can)

Preheat oven to 375 degrees. In a small covered container, shake flour with 1/2 cup of broth.

In a medium skillet** that has been sprayed with nonstick cooking spray, add remaining broth, milk, and flour mixture.

Bring to a boil, stirring constantly until thickened. Reduce heat and add chicken, peas, mushrooms, pimiento, parsley, and pepper. Return to a boil, reduce heat and simmer, stirring occasionally, for 5 minutes.

In a 2-quart casserole** that has been sprayed with nonstick cooking spray, add hot chicken mixture.

Place biscuits on top of the hot chicken mixture. Bake 20 minutes or until biscuits are golden brown. Let set for 5 minutes before serving. Serve in bowls.

***If you have a skillet with an oven-proof handle, omit the 2-quart casserole and use the skillet in the oven.*

NOTE: One serving is a good source of fiber.

Sodium is figured for reduced sodium.

 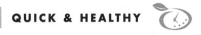

Chicken and Artichokes Dijon

Dijon sauce:
1/4 cup light mayonnaise
3 tablespoons fat-free plain yogurt
1 tablespoon Dijon mustard
2 teaspoons sugar or the equivalent in artificial sweetener
1 teaspoon dried parsley
1/4 teaspoon ground black pepper

1 cup uncooked quick-cooking brown rice
1 cup fat-free chicken broth*
1 pound skinless, boneless chicken breasts, cut into strips
1 cup chopped red bell pepper
1 can (14 ounces) quartered artichoke hearts, drained and rinsed

Preheat oven to 350 degrees. Mix mayonnaise, yogurt, mustard, sugar, and seasonings to make the sauce. Set aside.

Spread rice in the bottom of a 2-quart covered casserole that has been sprayed with nonstick cooking spray. Pour broth over rice. Arrange chicken and vegetables over rice. Cover and bake for 45 minutes.

Top with sauce. Return to oven, uncovered, for 5 minutes.

NOTE: One serving is an excellent source of fiber.

Sodium is figured for reduced sodium.

The rich-tasting Dijon sauce combined with the artichoke hearts gives a delightful flavor to this recipe. It's a good choice for company.

Makes 4 servings

Each Serving

Carb Servings
2

Exchanges
1 1/2 starch
1 vegetable
4 lean meat

Nutrient Analysis
calories 316—with artificial sweetener 308
total fat 7g
saturated fat 1g
cholesterol 70mg
sodium 471mg
total carbohydrate 28g—with artificial sweetener 26g
dietary fiber 5g
sugars 5g—with artificial sweetener 3g
protein 31g

This recipe has a very good flavor and is a family pleaser. It only takes a few minutes to assemble, especially if you purchase cleaned baby carrots and celery stalks.

Makes 4 servings

Each Serving

Carb Servings
1 1/2

Exchanges
1 1/2 starch
1 vegetable
3 lean meat

Nutrient Analysis
calories 247
total fat 2g
saturated fat 0g
cholesterol 65mg
sodium 231mg
total carbohydrate 25g
dietary fiber 4g
sugars 4g
protein 29g

Chicken and Rice Casserole

1 cup uncooked quick-cooking brown rice
1 pound skinless, boneless chicken breasts, cut into bite-size pieces
1 1/2 cups sliced carrots
1 cup sliced celery
1/2 cup chopped onion
1 cup fat-free chicken broth*
1 teaspoon chopped garlic
1 teaspoon Italian seasoning
1/4 teaspoon salt (optional)
1/8 teaspoon ground black pepper

Preheat oven to 350 degrees.

Spray a covered 2-quart casserole with nonstick cooking spray. Spread rice in the casserole. Top rice with chicken and vegetables.

Mix seasonings with broth. Pour over chicken mixture. Cover and bake for 45 minutes. Let set 10 minutes before serving.

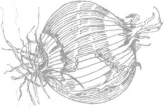

NOTE: One serving is a good source of fiber.

*Sodium is figured for reduced sodium.

Chicken Breasts in Mushroom Sauce

2 cups sliced mushrooms
1/4 cup chopped green onion
2 tablespoons unbleached all-purpose flour
1/4 cup water
1/2 cup fat-free plain yogurt
2 tablespoons dry sherry or water
1 teaspoon instant chicken bouillon*
1/4 teaspoon salt (optional)
1/8 teaspoon ground black pepper
1 pound skinless, boneless chicken breasts
1/4 teaspoon paprika

Preheat oven to 350 degrees. Sauté mushrooms and onion in a skillet that has been sprayed with a nonstick cooking spray.

Meanwhile, mix flour and water in a covered container and shake well to prevent lumps. Add to mushrooms along with next five ingredients. Cook, stirring constantly, until thickened.

Arrange chicken in a 9-inch by 9-inch baking dish that has been sprayed with nonstick cooking spray. Pour mushroom sauce over chicken and sprinkle with paprika. Bake for 30 minutes or until chicken is no longer pink.

Sodium is figured for reduced sodium.

The sherry and yogurt add a good flavor to this recipe. The sauce is good over brown rice, potatoes, or noodles.

Makes 4 servings

Each Serving

Carb Servings
1/2

Exchanges
1/2 carbohydrate
3 lean meat

Nutrient Analysis
calories 170
total fat 2g
saturated fat 0g
cholesterol 66mg
sodium 152mg
total carbohydrate 8g
dietary fiber 1g
sugars 3g
protein 29g

Makes 6 servings

Each Serving

Carb Servings
0

Exchanges
3 lean meat

Nutrient Analysis
calories 137
total fat 1g
saturated fat 0g
cholesterol 65mg
sodium 100mg
total carbohydrate 3g
dietary fiber 0g
sugars 0g
protein 26g

Oven-Fried Chicken

1/4 cup cornflake crumbs
1/4 teaspoon dried thyme
1/4 teaspoon dried sage
1/8 teaspoon salt (optional)
1/8 teaspoon ground black pepper
1 1/2 pounds skinless, boneless chicken breasts or
   2 1/2–3 pounds chicken parts

Preheat oven to 425 degrees. Skin chicken if parts are used. Spray a 9-inch by 13-inch baking pan with nonstick cooking spray.

Mix the first five ingredients in a plastic bag. Place a few pieces of chicken at a time in the plastic bag and shake to coat evenly.

Arrange chicken pieces in the pan so that they are not touching. Bake boneless chicken breasts for 15–20 minutes and chicken parts for 45–60 minutes.

VARIATION: *Italian Oven-Fried Chicken*—Substitute 1/2 teaspoon of Italian seasoning for the dried sage and dried thyme.

Chicken Nuggets

1/2 cup cornflake crumbs
1/2 teaspoon dried thyme
1/2 teaspoon dried sage
1/4 teaspoon salt (optional)
1/8 teaspoon ground black pepper
1 pound skinless, boneless chicken breasts
assorted mustards (optional)

Mix the first five ingredients in a plastic bag and set aside.

Cut chicken into bite-size pieces. Place a few pieces of chicken at a time in the plastic bag and shake to coat evenly. Follow directions below for microwave or conventional oven.

MICROWAVE OVEN: Arrange chicken pieces, so they are not touching, in a 9-inch by 13-inch glass baking dish that has been sprayed with nonstick cooking spray. Cover with wax paper and cook on high for 6–8 minutes or until chicken is cooked, rearranging twice during cooking time.

CONVENTIONAL OVEN: Preheat oven to 425 degrees. Arrange chicken pieces, so they are not touching, in a baking pan that has been sprayed with nonstick cooking spray. Bake for 12–14 minutes.

Optional mustards for dipping:
sweet and sour—25 calories per tablespoon
honey mustard—35 calories per tablespoon
hot mustard (prepared) or dry mustard (follow package directions to mix with water)—10 calories per tablespoon

VARIATION: *Italian Chicken Nuggets*—Substitute 1 teaspoon of Italian seasoning for the dried sage and dried thyme.

These are a favorite for children. Serve with the Low-Fat French Fries recipe in this book. You can find cornflake crumbs in the breadings section of the grocery store.

Makes 4 servings

Each Serving

Carb Servings
1/2

Exchanges
1/2 starch
3 lean meat

Nutrient Analysis
calories 164
total fat 1g
saturated fat 0g
cholesterol 65mg
sodium 153mg
total carbohydrate 9g
dietary fiber 0g
sugars 1g
protein 27g

This is a special way to serve chicken. It is so moist and flavorful. You can find cornflake crumbs in the breadings section of the grocery store.

Makes 8 servings

Each Serving

Carb Servings
1/2

Exchanges
1/2 starch
3 lean meat

Nutrient Analysis
calories 162
total fat 1g
saturated fat 0g
cholesterol 65mg
sodium 138mg
total carbohydrate 6g
dietary fiber 0g
sugars 1g
protein 27g

Chicken Breasts Supreme

1/2 cup cornflake crumbs
1/2 teaspoon dried thyme
1/2 teaspoon dried sage
1/4 teaspoon salt (optional)
1/8 teaspoon ground black pepper
2 pounds skinless, boneless chicken breasts
1/2 cup sliced onion
1/2 cup fat-free chicken broth*
1/2 cup dry white wine, vermouth, or chicken broth
2 cups mushrooms, sliced

Preheat oven to 375 degrees. Mix the first five ingredients in a plastic bag. Place a couple pieces of chicken at a time in the plastic bag and shake to coat evenly. Arrange chicken in a 9-inch by 13-inch baking pan that has been sprayed with nonstick cooking spray.

Spray a skillet with nonstick cooking spray and sauté onions. Add broth and wine. Bring to a boil. Pour around chicken.

Bake, uncovered, for 30 minutes.

Meanwhile, in the same skillet, sauté mushrooms. Arrange mushrooms around chicken after the chicken has cooked for 30 minutes. Bake an additional 10 minutes or until chicken is no longer pink.

*Sodium is figured for reduced sodium.

Crispy Potato Chicken

1 pound skinless, boneless chicken breasts
2 tablespoons Dijon mustard
1/2 teaspoon chopped garlic
2 new potatoes, not peeled (about 5 ounces, total)
1 teaspoon oil (canola or olive)
1/4 teaspoon lemon juice*
1 teaspoon ground black pepper

Preheat oven to 425 degrees. Arrange chicken in a 9-inch by 9-inch baking dish that has been sprayed with nonstick cooking spray.

Mix mustard and garlic. Spread over chicken.

Grate potatoes and mix with oil and lemon juice. Spread over chicken. Sprinkle with pepper. Bake for 25–35 minutes until chicken is no longer pink and potatoes are golden brown.

Lemon juice is used to prevent the potatoes from turning gray.

Makes 4 servings

Each Serving

Carb Servings
1/2

Exchanges
1/2 starch
3 lean meat

Nutrient Analysis
calories 167
total fat 3g
saturated fat 0g
cholesterol 65mg
sodium 255mg
total carbohydrate 6g
dietary fiber 1g
sugars 0g
protein 27g

The combination of cumin, yogurt, and jam makes this a flavorful dish.

Makes 4 servings

Each Serving

Carb Servings
0

Exchanges
3 lean meat

Nutrient Analysis
calories 143
total fat 2g
saturated fat 0g
cholesterol 65mg
sodium 89mg
total carbohydrate 5g
dietary fiber 0g
sugars 1g
protein 27g

Yogurt Cumin Chicken

1 pound skinless, boneless chicken breasts
1/3 cup fat-free plain yogurt
3 tablespoons sugar-free apricot preserves
1 teaspoon ground cumin
1/2 teaspoon salt (optional)

Choose from one of the three methods below for cooking.

CONVENTIONAL OVEN: Preheat oven to 350 degrees. Arrange chicken in a baking pan that has been sprayed with nonstick cooking spray. Bake, uncovered, for 20 minutes. Drain any liquid. Mix remaining ingredients and spoon over chicken. Bake for 10 minutes or until chicken is no longer pink and sauce is heated.

MICROWAVE OVEN: Arrange chicken in a microwave-safe dish. Cover with plastic wrap, venting one corner. Cook on high for 6–8 minutes, or until chicken is no longer pink, rotating 1/4 turn halfway through cooking time. Drain any liquid. Mix remaining ingredients and spoon over chicken. Cook for 1–2 minutes or until sauce is heated.

BROILER OR BARBECUE METHOD: Cut 3 shallow slits length-wise in each chicken breast half. Place slit side down on broiler pan. Mix remaining ingredients. Spoon half on chicken. Broil 3–4 inches from heat for 4 minutes. Turn chicken over and spoon on remaining yogurt mixture. Broil 5 minutes longer or until chicken is no longer pink.

French Glazed Chicken

1/4 cup fat-free French dressing
2 tablespoons sugar-free apricot preserves
2 tablespoons water
1 tablespoon dried or 1/4 cup fresh minced onion
1 pound skinless, boneless chicken breasts

Mix the first four ingredients and set aside.

Arrange chicken in a 9-inch by 9-inch baking pan that has been sprayed with nonstick cooking spray. Use a microwave-safe dish if cooking in the microwave. Follow directions below for microwave or conventional oven.

CONVENTIONAL OVEN: Preheat oven to 350 degrees. Bake, uncovered, for 20 minutes. Drain any liquid. Spoon apricot mixture over chicken. Return to oven for 10 minutes or until chicken is no longer pink and glaze is heated.

MICROWAVE OVEN: Cover with plastic wrap, venting one corner. Cook on high for 6–8 minutes, or until chicken is no longer pink. Rotate 1/4 turn halfway through cooking. Drain any liquid. Spoon apricot mixture over chicken. Cook for 1–2 minutes or until glaze is heated.

The orange glaze adds color as well as flavor to the chicken. This same glaze is used in French Glazed Fish.

Makes 4 servings

Each Serving

Carb Servings
1/2

Exchanges
1/2 carbohydrate
3 lean meat

Nutrient Analysis
calories 155
total fat 1g
saturated fat 0g
cholesterol 65mg
sodium 223mg
total carbohydrate 9g
dietary fiber 0g
sugars 3g
protein 26g

This attractive dish is so easy to assemble and looks so impressive. It is good served hot or cold. When preparing the asparagus, snap off the fibrous end and soak the tips in water to remove any dirt.

Makes 4 servings

Each Serving

Carb Servings
1/2

Exchanges
1 vegetable
3 lean meat

Nutrient Analysis
calories 151
total fat 2g
saturated fat 0g
cholesterol 65mg
sodium 82mg
total carbohydrate 6g
dietary fiber 3g
sugars 2g
protein 28g

Rolled Chicken and Asparagus

1 pound skinless, boneless chicken breasts
24–30 asparagus spears (tough ends removed)
2 tablespoons lemon juice
6 green onions, chopped
1/2 teaspoon salt (optional)
1/2 teaspoon ground black pepper

Preheat oven to 350 degrees. Cut chicken breasts into 8 or 10 strips, each about 1 inch by 5 inches long.

Wrap each strip in a corkscrew fashion around 2 or 3 uncooked asparagus spears. Fasten with toothpicks. Place in a covered baking dish that has been sprayed with nonstick cooking spray. Sprinkle with lemon juice, green onions, salt, and pepper.

Cover and bake 25–30 minutes or until chicken is no longer pink. Remove toothpicks. Serve hot or refrigerate until chilled and serve cold.

NOTE: One serving is a good source of fiber.

Chicken Picadillo

1 pound skinless, boneless chicken breasts
1 teaspoon ground cumin
3/4 cup salsa, thick and chunky
1/2 teaspoon chopped garlic
1 medium onion, sliced
1 medium green pepper, sliced

Cut chicken into 1-inch strips. Sprinkle with cumin.

Spray skillet with nonstick cooking spray. Stir-fry chicken until tender and no longer pink. Add salsa, garlic, onion, and green pepper.

Cover and simmer for 10 minutes or until vegetables are tender.

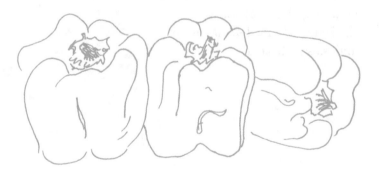

Serve this in a whole-wheat tortilla or with a whole-grain roll. It is also good served with brown rice. To reduce the sodium, use the salsa recipe in this book.

Makes 4 servings

Each Serving

Carb Servings
1/2

Exchanges
2 vegetable
3 lean meat

Nutrient Analysis
calories 165
total fat 2g
saturated fat 0g
cholesterol 65mg
sodium 297mg
total carbohydrate 9g
dietary fiber 1g
sugars 4g
protein 27g

Makes 4 servings

Each Serving

Carb Servings
0

Exchanges
3 lean meat

Nutrient Analysis
calories 138
total fat 1g
saturated fat 0g
cholesterol 65mg
sodium 293mg
total carbohydrate 3g
dietary fiber 0g
sugars 2g
protein 26g

Chicken in Salsa

1 pound skinless, boneless chicken breasts
3/4 cup salsa

Arrange chicken in a 9-inch by 9-inch baking pan that has been sprayed with nonstick cooking spray. Use a microwave-safe dish if cooking in the microwave. Follow directions below for microwave or conventional oven.

CONVENTIONAL OVEN: Preheat oven to 350 degrees. Bake, uncovered, for 20 minutes. Spoon salsa over chicken. Return to oven for 10 minutes or until chicken is no longer pink and salsa is heated.

MICROWAVE OVEN: Cover with plastic wrap, venting one corner. Cook on high for 6–8 minutes, or until chicken is no longer pink. Rotate 1/4 turn halfway through cooking time. Drain any liquid. Spoon salsa over chicken. Cook for 1–2 minutes or until salsa is heated.

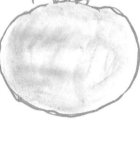

Chicken Fajitas

3 tablespoons lime juice
1/2 teaspoon dried cilantro
1/2 teaspoon chili powder
1 pound skinless, boneless chicken breasts, cut into
    1-inch strips
1 medium green pepper, sliced
1 medium onion, sliced
4 (8-inch) or 8 (6-inch) whole-wheat tortillas
salsa (optional)

Mix lime juice with coriander and chili powder. Pour over chicken. Add sliced vegetables.

Spray skillet with nonstick cooking spray. Stir-fry chicken and vegetables until chicken is no longer pink and vegetables are crisp-tender.

Warm tortillas in microwave about 50 seconds on high or in a nonstick skillet. Fill each tortilla with chicken mixture and serve with salsa and fat-free sour cream or fat-free yogurt.

NOTE: One serving is a good source of fiber.

This is a good family recipe. Serve with fat-free refried beans.

Makes 4 servings

Each Serving

Carb Servings
2

Exchanges
1 1/2 starch
1 vegetable
3 lean meat

Nutrient Analysis
calories 278
total fat 3g
saturated fat 0g
cholesterol 65mg
sodium 280mg
total carbohydrate 30g
dietary fiber 3g
sugars 6g
protein 32g

This is a favorite for those of us who like Mexican food. Sodium is figured for bottled salsa. To reduce the sodium, use the salsa recipe in this book.

Makes 4 servings

Each Serving

Carb Servings
2

Exchanges
1 1/2 starch
1 vegetable
3 lean meat

Nutrient Analysis
calories 260
total fat 5g
saturated fat 2g
cholesterol 50mg
sodium 544mg
total carbohydrate 27g
dietary fiber 2g
sugars 5g
protein 24g

Baked Chimichangas

4 (8-inch) or 8 (6-inch) whole-wheat tortillas

Filling:
1 1/2 cups cooked and cubed chicken
3/4 cup salsa, thick and chunky
1/2 cup (2 ounces) grated, reduced-fat cheddar or Mexican blend cheese

Optional:
extra salsa
Spanish Yogurt Sauce (page 122)

Preheat oven to 400 degrees. Mix filling ingredients in a medium bowl.

Warm tortillas until pliable (about 5 seconds each in microwave or in a nonstick skillet). Wet one side of tortilla and place wet side down. Spoon on filling ingredients. Fold to hold in filling.

Spray baking dish with nonstick cooking spray. Lay chimichangas, seam side down, on baking dish. Bake for 15 minutes.

VARIATIONS: *Beef, Pork, or Turkey Chimichangas*–Substitute ground or diced beef, pork, or turkey for chicken.

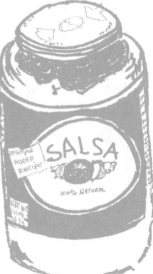

Chicken Tortilla Casserole

2 cans (10.75 ounces each) low-fat, condensed cream of chicken soup*

1 can of water

1 can (7 ounces) diced green chiles

1/4 cup dried or 1 cup fresh minced onion

1 teaspoon ground cumin

1/2 teaspoon chili powder

9 whole-wheat tortillas (8-inch), cut into 1-inch strips

4 cups cooked and cubed chicken

1 cup (4 ounces) grated, reduced-fat cheddar cheese

Preheat oven to 350 degrees. Spray a 9-inch by 13-inch baking pan with nonstick cooking spray.

Combine soup with water. Add the next four ingredients and set aside.

Place 1/3 of the tortilla strips in the pan. Top with 1/2 the chicken, 1/3 of the soup mixture. Repeat layering with 1/3 of the tortilla strips, remaining chicken, 1/3 of the soup mixture, remaining tortillas, and remaining soup mixture. Bake uncovered for 35–40 minutes. Top with cheese and bake for another 5 minutes.

NOTE: One serving is a good source of fiber.

Sodium is figured for reduced sodium.

This is a popular dish to take to potlucks. It is also a good way to use leftover chicken or turkey. Serve it with salsa or the Spanish Yogurt Sauce recipe in this book.

Makes 10 servings

Each Serving

Carb Servings
2

Exchanges
2 starch
3 lean meat

Nutrient Analysis
calories 274
total fat 6g
saturated fat 2g
cholesterol 55mg
sodium 570mg
total carbohydrate 30g
dietary fiber 3g
sugars 4g
protein 25g

Makes 8 servings

Each Serving

Carb Servings
2

Exchanges
1 starch
2 vegetable
3 lean meat

Nutrient Analysis
calories 281
total fat 8g
saturated fat 2g
cholesterol 63mg
sodium 822mg
total carbohydrate 27g
dietary fiber 2g
sugars 4g
protein 27g

Green Chile Chicken Enchilada Casserole

1 can (28 ounces) green chile enchilada sauce, divided
4 cups cooked and cubed chicken
1/2 cup fat-free sour cream
1 can (7 ounces) diced green chiles
1/4 cup dried or 1 cup fresh minced onions
1 cup (4 ounces) grated, reduced-fat cheddar or Mexican cheese, divided
12 corn tortillas (6-inch)

Preheat oven to 350 degrees. Spray a 9-inch by 13-inch baking pan with nonstick cooking spray.

Combine 1 1/2 cups of enchilada sauce with chicken, sour cream, chiles, onions, and 1/2 cup of grated cheese. Set aside.

Place 1/3 of the tortillas in the pan, tearing tortillas to fill any empty areas. Top with 1/2 of the chicken mixture. Add another layer of the tortillas, top with remaining chicken mixture and remaining tortillas. Pour remaining enchilada sauce over all. Bake uncovered for 40 minutes. Top with remaining grated cheese and return to oven for 5 minutes.

NOTE: This recipe is higher in sodium and should be limited by those on a low-sodium diet.

Chicken Enchiladas

2 cups cooked and cubed chicken
1 cup chopped onion
1 cup low-fat cottage cheese or Ricotta cheese
1 cup fat-free plain yogurt
1/2 cup (2 ounces) grated, reduced-fat cheddar or
    Mexican blend cheese
1/2 cup (2 ounces) grated, reduced-fat mozzarella cheese
2 cans (10 ounces each) enchilada sauce, divided
12 corn tortillas (6-inch)

Preheat oven to 375 degrees. Mix the first six ingredients
and set aside.

Spray a 9-inch by 13-inch baking dish with nonstick
cooking spray. Pour 1/2 can of enchilada sauce in bottom
of pan. Follow either method below for layered or rolled.
Then bake for 20–30 minutes or until heated thoroughly.

ROLLED METHOD: Place about 1/3 to 1/2 cup of filling
on each tortilla and roll to enclose (cracks in tortillas are
not as noticeable after cooking). Place seam side down in
baking dish. Top with remaining sauce.

LAYERED METHOD: Layer in this order: 1/3 of the
tortillas, 1/2 of the filling, 1/3 tortillas, 1 can of sauce,
remainder of filling, remainder of tortillas, remainder
of sauce.

VARIATIONS: *Turkey, Pork, or Beef Enchiladas*–Substitute 2
cups of ground or shredded meat for the chicken.

NOTE: One serving is a good source of fiber.

This recipe is higher in sodium and should be limited by
those on a low-sodium diet.

This recipe can be layered to save time or you can fill each tortilla and roll in the traditional way. Turkey, pork, or beef can be substituted for the chicken.

Makes 8 servings

Each Serving

Carb Servings
2

Exchanges
1 1/2 starch
1 vegetable
2 lean meat

Nutrient Analysis
calories 237
total fat 6g
saturated fat 2g
cholesterol 40mg
sodium 757mg
total carbohydrate 26g
dietary fiber 3g
sugars 4g
protein 19g

The flavor of the coconut milk combined with fresh ginger and cilantro makes this Asian dish especially delicious. Light coconut milk has 60% less calories and fat than regular coconut milk, however it is high in saturated fat and should be limited. If you like spicy-hot dishes, add the fresh chili paste. Brown rice can be substituted for pasta.

Grilled Chicken with Coconut-Cilantro Sauce

3/4 cup light coconut milk*
2 sliced green onions
1 1/2 tablespoons minced fresh ginger
1 tablespoon lite soy sauce
1 tablespoon brown sugar or the equivalent in artificial sweetener
1 tablespoon lime juice
1 teaspoon chopped garlic
1/2 teaspoon ground fresh chili paste* (optional)
4 ounces of uncooked pasta
1 pound skinless, boneless chicken breasts, cut into strips
1/2 cup chopped fresh cilantro

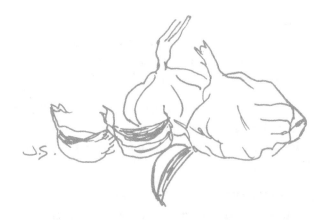

In a small saucepan combine the first eight ingredients. Simmer for 5 minutes.

Meanwhile, cook pasta according to package direction. Drain and keep warm, according to package directions.

BARBECUE: When barbecue is hot, place chicken on grill. Spoon a couple of tablespoons of coconut sauce over chicken. Cook about 4 minutes on each side or until chicken is no longer pink.

CONVENTIONAL OVEN: Preheat oven to 350 degrees. Place chicken in a 9-inch by 13-inch baking pan that has been sprayed with nonstick cooking spray. Spoon a couple of tablespoons of coconut sauce over chicken. Bake for 20–30 minutes or until chicken is no longer pink.

Add fresh cilantro to the sauce just before serving. Serve chicken with warm coconut-cilantro sauce and pasta.

Found in the Asian section of the grocery store.

When buying a 13-ounce can of coconut milk, use half and freeze the remainder for another meal. Coconut milk is also used in Grilled Salmon with Coconut-Cilantro Sauce.

Makes 5 servings

Each Serving

Carb Servings
1 1/2—with artificial sweetener 1

Exchanges
1 vegetable
1 starch
3 lean meat

Nutrient Analysis
calories 226—with artificial sweetener 216
total fat 4g
saturated fat 2g
cholesterol 52mg
sodium 185mg
total carbohydrate 23g—with artificial sweetener 19g
dietary fiber 1g
sugars 4g—with artificial sweetener 2g
protein 25g

This is another complete meal in a pot. Serve with a dollop of fat-free yogurt or fat-free sour cream.

Makes 5 servings

Each Serving

Carb Servings
1 1/2

Exchanges
1 starch
2 vegetable
3 lean meat

Nutrient Analysis
calories 241
total fat 4g
saturated fat 2g
cholesterol 59mg
sodium 221mg
total carbohydrate 25g
dietary fiber 3g
sugars 6g
protein 27g

Mexican-Style Chicken and Rice

1 cup uncooked quick-cooking brown rice
1 pound skinless, boneless chicken breasts, cut into bite-size pieces
1 medium onion, chopped (about 1 cup)
1 medium green pepper, chopped (about 1 cup)
1 can (14.5 ounces) diced tomatoes*, not drained
1 can (4 ounces) diced green chiles
1/2 cup water
1 teaspoon chopped garlic
1/2 teaspoon ground cumin
3 drops Tabasco sauce
1/4 teaspoon salt (optional)
1/8 teaspoon ground black pepper
1/2 cup (2 ounces) grated, reduced-fat cheddar cheese or reduced-fat Mexican cheese

Preheat oven to 350 degrees. Spray a covered 2-quart casserole with nonstick cooking spray.

Spread rice in the casserole. Top with chicken, onion, and green pepper. Mix tomatoes, chiles, water, and seasonings. Pour over chicken mixture.

Cover and bake for 45 minutes. Top with cheese and return to oven for 5 minutes or until cheese is melted.

NOTE: One serving is a good source of fiber.

Sodium is figured for no added salt.

 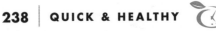

Grilled Chicken with Corn Salsa

This is a great recipe for a summer barbecue but can also be prepared in the oven. This salsa is especially flavorful.

Corn Salsa
1 can (14.5 ounces) diced tomatoes*, not drained, or
  1 1/2 cups chopped fresh tomato
2/3 cup frozen whole-kernel corn
1 cup chopped cucumber, not peeled
1/2 cup chopped bell pepper, red or green
1/4 cup chopped fresh cilantro
2 tablespoons red wine vinegar
1/2 teaspoon each: garlic powder and ground cumin
1/4 teaspoon salt (optional)
1/8 teaspoon ground black pepper
1/8 teaspoon cayenne pepper

2 pounds skinless, boneless chicken breasts, cut into strips
1/4 teaspoon salt (optional)
1/8 teaspoon ground black pepper

Combine salsa ingredients and set aside.

BARBECUE: When barbecue is hot, place chicken on grill. Season with salt and pepper. Cook about 4 minutes on each side or until chicken is no longer pink.

CONVENTIONAL OVEN: Preheat oven to 350 degrees. Place chicken in a 9-inch by 13-inch baking pan that has been sprayed with nonstick cooking spray. Season with salt and pepper. Bake for 20–30 minutes or until chicken is no longer pink.

Serve chicken topped with corn salsa.

Sodium is figured for no added salt.

Makes 8 servings
4 cups salsa plus chicken

Each Serving
1/2 cup salsa plus 1/8
  chicken

Carb Servings
1/2

Exchanges
1 vegetable
3 lean meat

Nutrient Analysis
calories 152
total fat 2g
saturated fat 0g
cholesterol 65mg
sodium 82mg
total carbohydrate 6g
dietary fiber 1g
sugars 4g
protein 27g

Makes 4 servings
4 cups salsa plus chicken

Each Serving
1 cup salsa plus 1/4 chicken

Carb Servings
1

Exchanges
1 fruit
4 lean meat

Nutrient Analysis
calories 230
total fat 8g
saturated fat 1g
cholesterol 65mg
sodium 84mg
total carbohydrate 13g
dietary fiber 5g
sugars 5g
protein 27g

Grilled Chicken with Fruit Salsa

Fruit Salsa
2 tablespoons lime juice
1 avocado, peeled, pitted and chopped
2 cups cubed fresh fruit such as red papaya, nectarine, apricot, or peaches
4 green onions, chopped
1/2 cup chopped fresh cilantro
1/2 teaspoon chopped garlic
1/4 teaspoon salt (optional)
1/8 teaspoon ground black pepper

1 pound skinless, boneless chicken breasts, cut into strips
1/4 teaspoon salt (optional)
1/8 teaspoon ground black pepper

Pour lime juice over avocado to prevent browning. Mix with remaining salsa ingredients and set aside. Serve over cooked chicken.

BARBECUE: When barbecue is hot, place chicken on grill. Season with salt and pepper. Cook about 4 minutes on each side or until chicken is no longer pink.

CONVENTIONAL OVEN: Preheat oven to 350 degrees. Place chicken in a 9-inch by 9-inch baking pan that has been sprayed with nonstick cooking spray. Season with salt and pepper. Bake for 20–30 minutes or until chicken is no longer pink.

NOTE: One serving is an excellent source of fiber.

Most of the fat in this recipe is heart-healthy monounsaturated fat.

Hickory-Smoked Barbecued Chicken

1 pound skinless, boneless chicken breasts or 2 pounds chicken parts
1/4 cup fat-free chicken broth*, or white wine
2 tablespoons lite soy sauce
2 tablespoons water
1 teaspoon hickory liquid smoke**
1/2 teaspoon ground ginger

Skin chicken if parts are used. Mix the remaining ingredients. Add chicken and marinate in the refrigerator for 1–3 hours. Drain and discard marinade. Use one of the methods below for cooking.

BARBECUE: When barbecue is hot, place chicken on grill. Cook about 4 minutes on each side or until chicken is no longer pink.

BROIL: Preheat oven to broil. Place chicken on broiler pan that has been sprayed with nonstick cooking spray. Cook about 4 minutes on each side or until chicken is no longer pink.

CONVENTIONAL OVEN: Preheat oven to 350 degrees. Place chicken in a 9-inch by 13-inch baking pan that has been sprayed with nonstick cooking spray. Bake for 20–30 minutes or until chicken is no longer pink.

Sodium is figured for reduced sodium.

**Hickory liquid smoke can be found in the grocery store next to the barbecue sauce.*

This is best barbecued but can be broiled or baked. The hickory liquid smoke gives this dish an excellent flavor.

Makes 4 servings

Each Serving

Carb Servings
0

Exchanges
3 lean meat

Nutrient Analysis
calories 127
total fat 1g
saturated fat 0g
cholesterol 65mg
sodium 231mg
total carbohydrate 0g
dietary fiber 0g
sugars 0g
protein 26g

This recipe has a light cornstarch gravy. It is especially good if you stir-fry the vegetables so that they are still crisp. Fresh broccoli can be substituted for the fresh pea pods.

Makes 4 servings

Each Serving

Carb Servings
1

Exchanges
3 vegetable
3 lean meat

Nutrient Analysis
calories 188
total fat 2g
saturated fat 0g
cholesterol 65mg
sodium 344mg
total carbohydrate 14g
dietary fiber 4g
sugars 5g
protein 28g

Chicken and Pea Pod Stir-Fry

1 pound skinless, boneless chicken breasts
1/2 cup cold water
2 tablespoons dry sherry or water (optional)
1 1/2 tablespoons lite soy sauce
1 tablespoon cornstarch
1 tablespoon chopped garlic
3 carrots, sliced diagonally
2 cups fresh snow pea pods
4 green onions, sliced

Cut chicken into bite-size pieces. Set aside. In a small bowl, combine water, sherry, soy sauce, cornstarch, and garlic. Set aside.

Spray a large skillet with nonstick cooking spray. Stir-fry chicken until no longer pink. Set aside and keep warm.

Add carrots to skillet and stir-fry for 3–5 minutes, adding water or broth, as needed, to prevent sticking. Add pea pods and onions. Stir-fry 2 minutes or until vegetables are crisp tender. Remove vegetables and keep warm.

Pour cornstarch mixture into skillet and stir until thickened and bubbly. Add vegetables and chicken. Cover and cook 1 minute.

NOTE: One serving is a good source of fiber.

 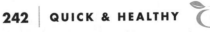

Spicy Chicken and Grapes

1 tablespoon cornstarch
3/4 cup fat-free chicken broth*, divided
2 tablespoons lite soy sauce
1 tablespoon granulated sugar or the equivalent in
artificial sweetener
1 tablespoon red wine vinegar
1–2 teaspoons ground fresh chili paste** (optional)
1 pound skinless, boneless chicken breasts, cut into
bite-size pieces
3 tablespoons fresh minced ginger
1 tablespoon chopped garlic
2 cups broccoli florets
1 1/2 cups green seedless grapes
3/4 cup thinly sliced green onions
1/4–1/2 cup fresh cilantro (optional)

In a small bowl, combine cornstarch and 1/4 cup chicken
broth. Add soy sauce, sugar, vinegar, and chili paste. Set
aside.

Spray a skillet with nonstick cooking spray. Add chicken,
ginger, and garlic. Stir-fry until chicken is no longer pink.
Remove from skillet and keep warm.

Add broccoli to skillet and stir-fry until crisp tender,
adding water or broth, as needed, to prevent sticking. Add
grapes, green onions, and the sauce mixture to the skillet.
Bring to a boil, stirring constantly for 1–2 minutes or until
thickened. Mix in cooked chicken. Top with cilantro just
before serving.

Sodium is figured for reduced sodium.

**Found in the Asian section of the grocery store.*

*Fresh cilantro and fresh
ginger are especially good
in this recipe. The chili
paste is spicy-hot, so use
cautiously or omit if you
don't like spicy foods.*

Makes 5 cups
5 servings

Each Serving
1 cup

Carb Servings
1

Exchanges
1 fruit
1 vegetable
3 lean meat

Nutrient Analysis
calories 172—with
artificial sweetener 162
total fat 1g
saturated fat 0g
cholesterol 52mg
sodium 383mg
total carbohydrate 17g—
with artificial sweetener
15g
dietary fiber 2g
sugars 11g—with artificial
sweetener 9g
protein 23g

Makes 5 cups
5 servings

Each Serving
1 cup

Carb Servings
1 1/2—with artificial
  sweetener 1

Exchanges
1 fruit—1/2 with artificial
  sweetener
1 vegetable
3 lean meat

Nutrient Analysis
calories 193—with
  artificial sweetener 152
total fat 1g
saturated fat 0g
cholesterol 52mg
sodium 239mg
total carbohydrate 23g—
  with artificial sweetener
  12g
dietary fiber 2g
sugars 16g—with artificial
  sweetener 5g
protein 22g

Sweet and Sour Chicken

1 can (8 ounces) unsweetened pineapple chunks, in juice
1 pound skinless, boneless chicken breasts
1 cup fat-free chicken broth*
1/4 cup cider vinegar
1/4 cup brown sugar or the equivalent in artificial
  sweetener**
2 teaspoons lite soy sauce
1/2 teaspoon chopped garlic
1 cup sliced celery
1 medium green pepper, sliced
1 small onion, quartered
3 tablespoons cornstarch
1/4 cup water

Drain pineapple, reserving the juice.

Cut chicken into bite-size pieces and place in a medium saucepan. Add reserved pineapple juice, broth, vinegar, brown sugar, soy sauce, and garlic. Cover and simmer over low heat for 15 minutes. Add vegetables and pineapple. Cook 10 minutes, stirring occasionally.

Combine cornstarch and water. Gradually stir into hot mixture. Continue to cook until thickened, stirring constantly.

Serve with brown rice.

Sodium is figured for reduced sodium.

**If using artificial sweetener, add after mixture is thickened with cornstarch.*

Teriyaki Chicken Stir-Fry

1 pound skinless, boneless chicken breasts, cut in
   bite-size pieces
1/4 cup teriyaki sauce
2 teaspoons chopped garlic
1 cup sliced red bell pepper
1 cup sliced green bell pepper
8 green onions, cut in 1-inch pieces
1/3 cup dry-roasted peanuts, unsalted

Combine chicken with teriyaki sauce and marinate for 1
hour in the refrigerator. Drain and discard marinade.

Spray a large skillet with nonstick cooking spray. Stir-
fry chicken with garlic until chicken is no longer pink.
Remove chicken from skillet and keep warm.

Add peppers and onion to skillet. Stir-fry a few minutes or
until vegetables are crisp-tender, adding water as needed
to prevent sticking. Add chicken and peanuts. Serve over
rice or noodles.

NOTE: One serving is a good source of fiber.

Most of the fat in this recipe is heart-healthy
monounsaturated fat.

*This is a great Oriental
stir-fry dish that is
colorful and delicious.*

Makes 6 cups
4 servings

Each Serving
1 1/2 cups

Carb Servings
1/2

Exchanges
2 vegetable
4 lean meat

Nutrient Analysis
calories 210
total fat 6g
saturated fat 1g
cholesterol 65mg
sodium 427mg
total carbohydrate 10g
dietary fiber 3g
sugars 4g
protein 30g

Seafood

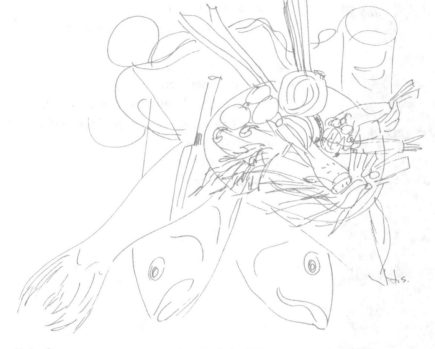

It is far too easy to overcook fish. The general rule is to cook 10 minutes for each inch of thickness. Fish should be cooked just until opaque and should flake easily with a fork.

The quality of frozen fish is usually very good, as it is often frozen within 4 hours of being caught. Look for frozen cooked shrimp in place of canned. It has a better flavor and is lower in sodium.

The flavor of the coconut milk combined with fresh ginger and cilantro makes this Asian dish especially delicious. Light coconut milk has 60% less calories and fat than regular coconut milk, however it is high in saturated fat and should be limited. If you like spicy-hot dishes, add the fresh chili paste. Serve with either potatoes, pasta, or rice.

Grilled Salmon with Coconut-Cilantro Sauce

3/4 cup light coconut milk*

2 sliced green onions

1 1/2 tablespoons minced fresh ginger

1 tablespoon lite soy sauce

1 tablespoon brown sugar or the equivalent in artificial sweetener

1 tablespoon lime juice

1 teaspoon chopped garlic

1/2 teaspoon ground fresh chili paste* (optional)

4 cups sliced new potatoes (not peeled), or 3 cups cooked brown rice or pasta

1/2 cup chopped fresh cilantro

1 1/2 pounds salmon fillets

In a small saucepan, combine the first eight ingredients. Simmer for 5 minutes.

Meanwhile, prepare potatoes by simmering in water until tender. Drain and keep warm.

BARBECUE: Before starting barbecue, spray aluminum foil with nonstick cooking spray. Note: Nonstick cooking spray is flammable. Do not spray near open flame or heated surfaces. Place foil over rack, poking holes in several areas. Start barbecue. When hot, place fish on foil. Spoon a couple tablespoons of coconut sauce over fish. Cook about 4 minutes on each side or until salmon flakes easily.

OVEN METHOD: Preheat oven to 450 degrees. Arrange fish in a 9-inch by 13-inch baking pan that has been sprayed with nonstick cooking spray. Spoon a couple tablespoons of coconut sauce over fish. Bake for 4–5 minutes per half inch thickness of fish. Drain any liquid.

Add fresh cilantro to the sauce just before serving. Serve salmon with warm coconut-cilantro sauce and potatoes, pasta, or rice.

NOTE: This recipe is a good source of heart-healthy omega-3 fat.

Found in the Asian section of the grocery store.

When buying a 13-ounce can of coconut milk, use half and freeze the remainder for another meal. Coconut milk is also used in Grilled Chicken with Coconut-Cilantro Sauce.

Makes 7 servings

Each Serving

Carb Servings
1

Exchanges
1 starch
3 lean meat

Nutrient Analysis
calories 237—with
 artificial sweetener 229
total fat 8g
saturated fat 2g
cholesterol 53mg
sodium 139mg
total carbohydrate 19g—
 with artificial sweetener
 17g
dietary fiber 3g
sugars 4g—with artificial
 sweetener 2g
protein 22g

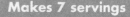

This is a great recipe for a summer barbecue but can also be prepared in the oven. This salsa is especially flavorful and colorful.

Grilled Salmon with Corn Salsa

Corn Salsa

1 can (14.5 ounces) diced tomatoes*, not drained, or
   1 1/2 cups chopped fresh tomato
2/3 cup frozen whole-kernel corn
1 cup chopped cucumber, not peeled
1/2 cup chopped bell pepper, red or green
1/4 cup chopped fresh cilantro
2 tablespoons red wine vinegar
1/2 teaspoon each: garlic powder and ground cumin
1/4 teaspoon salt (optional)
1/8 teaspoon ground black pepper
1/8 teaspoon cayenne pepper

2 pounds salmon fillets
1/4 teaspoon salt (optional)
1/8 teaspoon ground black pepper

Combine salsa ingredients and set aside.

Serve over cooked fish.

BARBECUE: Before starting barbecue, spray aluminum foil with nonstick cooking spray. *Note: Nonstick cooking spray is flammable. Do not spray near open flame or heated surfaces.* Place aluminum foil over rack, poking holes in several areas. Start barbecue. When hot, place fish on foil. Season with salt and pepper. Cook about 4 minutes on each side or until salmon flakes easily.

OVEN METHOD: Preheat oven to 450 degrees. Arrange fish in a 9-inch by 13-inch baking pan that has been sprayed with nonstick cooking spray. Season with salt and pepper. Bake, uncovered, for 4–5 minutes per half inch thickness of fish. Drain any liquid.

NOTE: This recipe is a good source of heart-healthy omega-3 fat.

*Sodium is figured for no added salt.

Makes 8 servings
4 cups salsa and fish for 8

Each Serving
1/2 cup salsa and 1/8 fish

Carb Servings
1/2

Exchanges
1 vegetable
3 lean meat

Nutrient Analysis
calories 189
total fat 7g
saturated fat 1g
cholesterol 62mg
sodium 59mg
total carbohydrate 6g
dietary fiber 1g
sugars 4g
protein 24g

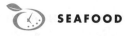

The fresh fruit salsa adds a unique taste to salmon. You can prepare the fish in your oven. However, the barbecue method is the best.

Grilled Salmon with Fruit Salsa

Fruit Salsa
1 avocado, peeled, pitted, and chopped
2 tablespoons lime juice
2 cups cubed fresh fruit such as red papaya, nectarine, apricot, or peaches
2 green onions, chopped
1/4 cup chopped fresh cilantro
1/2 teaspoon chopped garlic
1/4 teaspoon salt (optional)
1/8 teaspoon ground black pepper

1 pound salmon fillets
1/4 teaspoon salt (optional)
1/8 teaspoon ground black pepper

Combine salsa ingredients and set aside.

Serve over cooked fish.

BARBECUE: Before starting barbecue, spray aluminum foil with nonstick cooking spray. *Note: Nonstick cooking spray is flammable. Do not spray near open flame or heated surfaces.* Place aluminum foil over rack, poking holes in several areas. Start barbecue. When hot, place fish on foil. Season with salt and pepper. Cook about 4 minutes on each side or until salmon flakes easily.

CONVENTIONAL OVEN: Preheat oven to 450 degrees. Arrange fish in a 9-inch by 13-inch baking pan that has been sprayed with nonstick cooking spray. Season with salt and pepper. Bake, uncovered, for 4–5 minutes per half inch thickness of fish. Drain any liquid.

NOTE: One serving is an excellent source of fiber.

Most of the fat in this recipe is heart-healthy monounsaturated and omega-3 fat.

Makes 4 servings
4 cups of salsa and fish for 4

Each Serving
1 cup salsa and 1/4 fish

Carb Servings
1

Exchanges
1 fruit
3 lean meat
1 fat

Nutrient Analysis
calories 264
total fat 14g
saturated fat 2g
cholesterol 62mg
sodium 59mg
total carbohydrate 12g
dietary fiber 5g
sugars 5g
protein 24g

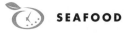

Makes 4 servings

Each Serving

Carb Servings
0

Exchanges
3 lean meat

Nutrient Analysis
calories 164
total fat 7g
saturated fat 1g
cholesterol 62mg
sodium 208mg
total carbohydrate 0g
dietary fiber 0g
sugars 0g
protein 23g

Hickory-Smoked Barbecued Fish

1/4 cup fat-free chicken broth*, or white wine
2 tablespoons lite soy sauce
2 tablespoons water
1 teaspoon hickory liquid smoke**
1/2 teaspoon ground ginger
1 pound firm fish such as salmon, snapper, or halibut

Mix the first five ingredients. Add fish and marinate in the refrigerator for 1–3 hours. Drain and discard marinade. Use one of the methods below for cooking.

BARBECUE: Before starting barbecue, spray aluminum foil with nonstick cooking spray. *Note: Nonstick cooking spray is flammable. Do not spray near open flame or heated surfaces.* Place aluminum foil over rack, poking holes in several areas. Start barbecue. When hot, place fish on foil. Cook about 4 minutes on each side or until fish flakes easily.

BROIL: Preheat oven to broil. Place fish on broiler pan that has been sprayed with nonstick cooking spray. Cook about 4 minutes on each side or until salmon flakes easily.

OVEN METHOD: Preheat oven to 450 degrees. Arrange fish in a 9-inch by 13-inch baking pan that has been sprayed with nonstick cooking spray. Bake, uncovered, for 4–5 minutes per half inch thickness of fish. Drain any liquid.

Sodium is figured for reduced sodium.

**Hickory liquid smoke can be found in the grocery store next to the barbecue sauce.*

 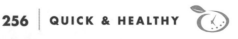

Polynesian Fish

1/4 cup fat-free chicken broth*, or white wine
2 tablespoons lite soy sauce
2 tablespoons water
1 teaspoon hickory liquid smoke**
1/2 teaspoon ground ginger
1 pound of firm fish such as salmon or snapper
1/4 cup brown sugar or the equivalent in artificial
  sweetener
1 teaspoon ground mustard

Mix the first five ingredients. Add fish and marinate in the refrigerator for 1–3 hours.

Preheat oven to 450 degrees.

Add fish and the marinade to a 9-inch by 13-inch baking pan that has been sprayed with nonstick cooking spray. Top fish pieces with 1/4 cup brown sugar and mustard. Bake, uncovered, for 4–5 minutes per half inch thickness of fish.

Pour sauce over fish when serving.

Sodium is figured for reduced sodium.

**Hickory liquid smoke can be found in the grocery store next to the barbecue sauce.*

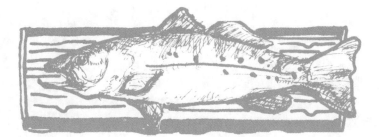

The hickory liquid smoke gives an excellent flavor to this recipe. The marinade becomes a delicious sauce that is especially good served over rice or noodles.

Makes 4 servings

Each Serving

Carb Servings
1—with artificial
  sweetener 0

Exchanges
1 carbohydrate—0 with
  artificial sweetener
3 lean meat

Nutrient Analysis
calories 223—with
  artificial sweetener 171
total fat 7g
saturated fat 1g
cholesterol 62mg
sodium 371mg
total carbohydrate 14g—
  with artificial sweetener
  1g
dietary fiber 0g
sugars 13g—with artificial
  sweetener 0g
protein 23g

This recipe is especially good with fresh red pepper, but a jar of pimentos will do. Leftover salmon is good to use and it is much lower in sodium than the canned red salmon.

Makes 4 servings

Each Serving
1 cake

Carb Servings
1/2

Exchanges
1/2 starch
2 lean meat
1 fat

Nutrient Analysis
calories 181
total fat 9g
saturated fat 2g
cholesterol 40mg
sodium 496mg
total carbohydrate 6g
dietary fiber 0g
sugars 2g
protein 18g

Salmon Cakes

1 can (14.75 ounces) red salmon, drained (or 2 cups flaked)
6 saltines (unsalted top), crushed
1/4 cup diced red pepper, or 1 jar (2 ounces) canned pimento
3 tablespoons Miracle Whip Light
1 teaspoon onion powder
1 teaspoon lemon juice
4 drops Tabasco sauce

Remove skin from fish and mash salmon bones with a fork, if using canned. Add saltines and red pepper.

Combine remaining ingredients. Add to salmon and mix well. Shape into 4 cakes.

Spray a skillet with nonstick cooking spray. Heat on medium. Cook salmon cakes, turning once, until lightly browned on each side.

NOTE: This recipe is a good source of heart-healthy omega-3 fat.

Cooking tip: Miracle Whip is preferred over mayonnaise, as it adds a touch of sweetness.

Oven-Fried Fish

1/4 cup cornflake crumbs*
1/2 teaspoon Italian seasoning
1/8 teaspoon salt (optional)
1/8 teaspoon ground black pepper
1 pound fish fillets (such as snapper, sole, halibut)

Preheat oven to 450 degrees. Spray a baking sheet with nonstick cooking spray. Mix the first four ingredients in a plastic bag and set aside.

Cut fish into serving size pieces. Place a few pieces of fish at a time in the plastic bag and shake to coat evenly.

Arrange on baking sheet so that fish is not touching. Bake for 10 minutes, per inch of thickness, or until fish flakes easily.

*You can find cornflake crumbs in the breadings section of the grocery store.

This is a healthy substitute for fried fish since it eliminates the cooking oil. Serve it with the Fresh Cucumber Sauce recipe in this book.

Makes 4 servings

Each Serving

Carb Servings
0

Exchanges
3 lean meat

Nutrient Analysis
calories 134
total fat 2g
saturated fat 0g
cholesterol 42mg
sodium 112mg
total carbohydrate 5g
dietary fiber 0g
sugars 1g
protein 24g

Use extra-small or small oysters when making this recipe. Serve them with seafood cocktail sauce or the Fresh Cucumber Sauce recipe in this book.

Makes 4 servings

Each Serving

Carb Servings
1

Exchanges
1 starch
1 lean meat

Nutrient Analysis
calories 110
total fat 2g
saturated fat 0g
cholesterol 43mg
sodium 170mg
total carbohydrate 13g
dietary fiber 0g
sugars 1g
protein 9g

Oven-Fried Oysters

1/2 cup cornflake crumbs*
1 teaspoon Italian seasoning
1/4 teaspoon salt (optional)
1/8 teaspoon ground black pepper
1 jar (16 ounces) oysters, drained

Preheat oven to 425 degrees. Spray a baking sheet with nonstick cooking spray.

Mix the first four ingredients in a plastic bag. Place oysters in the bag, a few at a time, and shake to coat. Arrange on baking sheet so oysters are not touching.

Bake for 10–15 minutes, depending on the size of the oysters.

*You can find cornflake crumbs in the breadings section of the grocery store.

Lemon Fish

1 pound fish fillets (snapper, sole)
4–6 lemon slices
1/4 cup fat-free chicken broth* or white wine
1/2 teaspoon fat-free butter-flavored sprinkles
1/8 teaspoon ground black pepper
1 tablespoon dried parsley

Arrange fish in a 9-inch by 13-inch baking pan that
has been sprayed with nonstick cooking spray. Use a
microwave-safe dish if cooking in the microwave. Top
with remaining ingredients.

Follow directions below for microwave or conventional
oven.

MICROWAVE OVEN: Cover with plastic wrap, venting
one corner. Cook on high for 5–8 minutes (depending on
thickness), rotating 1/4 turn halfway through cooking.
Fish is done when it flakes easily with a fork.

CONVENTIONAL OVEN: Preheat oven to 450 degrees.
Bake fish, uncovered, for 10 minutes
per inch of thickness, or until fish
flakes easily with a fork.

Sodium is figured for reduced sodium.

*This has a very good
flavor and is so easy
to prepare.*

Makes 4 servings

Each Serving

Carb Servings
0

Exchanges
3 lean meat

Nutrient Analysis
calories 116
total fat 2g
saturated fat 0g
cholesterol 42mg
sodium 120mg
total carbohydrate 1g
dietary fiber 0g
sugars 0g
protein 23g

Makes 4 servings

Each Serving

Carb Servings
1/2

Exchanges
1/2 carbohydrate
3 lean meat

Nutrient Analysis
calories 145
total fat 2g
saturated fat 0g
cholesterol 42mg
sodium 223mg
total carbohydrate 9g
dietary fiber 0g
sugars 3g
protein 23g

French Glazed Fish

1/4 cup fat-free French dressing
2 tablespoons sugar-free apricot preserves
2 tablespoons water
1 tablespoon dried or 1/4 cup fresh minced onion
1 pound fish fillets (snapper, sole)

Mix the first four ingredients and set aside.

Arrange fish in a 9-inch by 13-inch baking pan that has been sprayed with nonstick cooking spray. Use a microwave-safe dish if cooking in the microwave. Follow directions below for microwave or conventional oven.

CONVENTIONAL OVEN: Preheat oven to 450 degrees. Bake, uncovered, for 4–5 minutes per 1/2 inch thickness of fish. Drain any liquid. Spoon apricot mixture over fish. Return to oven for 2 minutes to heat sauce.

MICROWAVE OVEN: Cover with plastic wrap, venting one corner. Cook on high for 4–6 minutes, depending on thickness of fish. Rotate 1/4 turn halfway through cooking time. Drain any liquid. Spoon apricot mixture over fish. Cook for 1–2 minutes or until sauce is heated.

Fish in Salsa

1 pound fish fillets (snapper, sole)
3/4 cup salsa, thick and chunky

Arrange fish in a 9-inch by 13-inch baking pan that
has been sprayed with nonstick cooking spray. Use a
microwave-safe dish if cooking in the microwave. Follow
directions below for microwave or conventional oven.

CONVENTIONAL OVEN: Preheat oven to 450 degrees.
Bake, uncovered, for 4–6 minutes per 1/2 inch thickness.
Drain any liquid. Spoon salsa over fish. Return to oven
for 2 minutes to heat salsa.

MICROWAVE OVEN: Cover with
plastic wrap, venting one corner.
Cook on high for 4–6 minutes,
depending on thickness of
fish. Rotate 1/4 turn halfway
through cooking. Drain any
liquid. Spoon salsa over fish.
Cook for 1–2 minutes or until
salsa is heated.

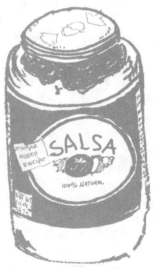

*This is a favorite for salsa
lovers. Sodium is figured
for bottled salsa. To reduce
the sodium, use the salsa
recipe in this book.*

Makes 4 servings

Each Serving

Carb Servings
0

Exchanges
3 lean meat

Nutrient Analysis
calories 128
total fat 2g
saturated fat 0g
cholesterol 42mg
sodium 293mg
total carbohydrate 3g
dietary fiber 0g
sugars 2g
protein 23g

Makes 4 servings

Each Serving

Carb Servings
1/2

Exchanges
1 vegetable
3 lean meat

Nutrient Analysis
calories 137
total fat 2g
saturated fat 0g
cholesterol 43mg
sodium 88mg
total carbohydrate 6g
dietary fiber 1g
sugars 3g
protein 24g

Spanish Baked Fish

1 pound fish fillets (snapper or sole)
1 can (8 ounces) tomato sauce*
1/2 cup sliced onions
1/2 teaspoon each: chopped garlic and chili powder
1/4 teaspoon each: dried oregano and ground cumin

Preheat oven to 450 degrees.

Arrange fish in a 9-inch by 13-inch baking pan that has been sprayed with nonstick cooking spray.

Mix remaining ingredients and pour over fish. Bake for 10–20 minutes or until fish flakes easily.

Sodium is figured for no added salt.

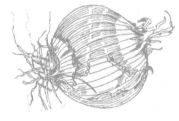

Poached Fish

1 cup fat-free chicken broth*
2 tablespoons lemon juice
1/2 teaspoon chopped garlic
1/4 teaspoon ground black pepper
2 bay leaves
2 tablespoons dry sherry (optional)
1 pound fish fillets (snapper, sole)

In a large skillet that has been sprayed with nonstick cooking spray, mix everything except fish. Bring to a boil. Reduce heat and add fish. Simmer, covered, for 3–5 minutes or until fish flakes easily.

Remove fish with slotted spatula. Discard bay leaves before serving.

Sodium is figured for reduced sodium.

This quick method for cooking fish also adds a good flavor.

Makes 4 servings

Each Serving

Carb Servings
0

Exchanges
3 lean meat

Nutrient Analysis
calories 120
total fat 2g
saturated fat 0g
cholesterol 42mg
sodium 169mg
total carbohydrate 1g
dietary fiber 0g
sugars 0g
protein 24g

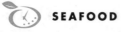

This sauce adds an interesting taste. Sodium is figured for bottled salsa. To reduce the sodium, prepare the salsa recipe in this book.

Makes 4 servings

Each Serving

Carb Servings
1—with artificial
    sweetener 0

Exchanges
1 carbohydrate—0 with
    artificial sweetener
3 lean meat

Nutrient Analysis
calories 162—with
    artificial sweetener 131
total fat 2g
saturated fat 0g
cholesterol 42mg
sodium 400mg
total carbohydrate 11g—
    with artificial sweetener
    2g
dietary fiber 0g
sugars 10g—with artificial
    sweetener 1g
protein 23g

Sweet Mustard Fish

1 pound fish fillets (snapper, sole)
1/2 cup salsa, thick and chunky
2 tablespoons honey or the equivalent in artificial
    sweetener
2 tablespoons Dijon mustard

Arrange fish in a 9-inch by 13-inch baking pan that has been sprayed with nonstick cooking spray. Use a microwave-safe dish if cooking in the microwave. Follow directions below for microwave or conventional oven.

CONVENTIONAL OVEN: Preheat oven to 450 degrees. Bake, uncovered, for 4–6 minutes per 1/2 inch thickness of fish. Drain any liquid. Combine remaining ingredients and spoon over fish. Return to oven for 2 minutes to heat sauce.

MICROWAVE OVEN: Cover with plastic wrap, venting one corner. Cook on high for 4–6 minutes, depending on thickness of fish. Rotate 1/4 turn halfway through cooking. Drain any liquid. Mix remaining ingredients and pour over fish. Cook for 1–2 minutes or until sauce is heated.

Tarragon Fish

1 pound fish fillets (snapper, sole)
1/2 cup fat-free plain yogurt
1 teaspoon dried tarragon
1/4 cup (1 ounce) grated, reduced-fat mozzarella cheese

Arrange fish in a 9-inch by 13-inch baking pan that has been sprayed with nonstick cooking spray. Use a microwave-safe dish if cooking in the microwave. Follow directions below for microwave or conventional oven.

CONVENTIONAL OVEN: Preheat oven to 450 degrees. Bake, uncovered, for 4–6 minutes per 1/2 inch thickness of fish. Drain any liquid. Mix remaining ingredients and spread over fish. Bake 2 minutes or until cheese is melted.

MICROWAVE OVEN: Cover with plastic wrap, venting one corner. Cook on high for 4–6 minutes, depending on thickness of fish. Rotate 1/4 turn halfway through cooking. Drain any liquid. Mix remaining ingredients and spread over fish. Cook for 1–2 minutes or until cheese is melted.

This recipe has a distinct tarragon flavor that is good with fish.

Makes 4 servings

Each Serving

Carb Servings
0

Exchanges
3 lean meat

Nutrient Analysis
calories 146
total fat 3g
saturated fat 1g
cholesterol 47mg
sodium 139mg
total carbohydrate 2g
dietary fiber 0g
sugars 2g
protein 26g

Yogurt Cumin Fish

This is a delicious way to serve fish when you're in a hurry. I like the combination of cumin with the sweetness of the apricot preserves.

Makes 4 servings

Each Serving

Carb Servings
0

Exchanges
3 lean meat

Nutrient Analysis
calories 132
total fat 2g
saturated fat 0g
cholesterol 42mg
sodium 88mg
total carbohydrate 5g
dietary fiber 0g
sugars 1g
protein 24g

1 pound fish fillets (snapper, sole)
1/3 cup fat-free plain yogurt
3 tablespoons sugar-free apricot preserves
1 teaspoon ground cumin
1/2 teaspoon salt (optional)

Arrange fish in a 9-inch by 13-inch baking pan that has been sprayed with nonstick cooking spray. Use a microwave-safe dish if cooking in the microwave. Follow directions below for microwave or conventional oven.

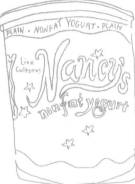

CONVENTIONAL OVEN: Preheat oven to 450 degrees. Bake, uncovered, for 4–5 minutes per 1/2 inch thickness of fish. Drain any liquid. Mix remaining ingredients and pour over fish. Bake for 2 minutes to heat sauce.

MICROWAVE OVEN: Cover with plastic wrap, venting one corner. Cook on high for 4–6 minutes, depending on thickness of fish. Rotate 1/4 turn halfway through cooking time. Drain any liquid. Mix remaining ingredients and pour over fish. Cook for 1–2 minutes or until sauce is heated.

Fillets of Sole Thermidor

2 pounds fillets of sole
1 teaspoon fat-free butter-flavored sprinkles
3/4 cup fat-free milk, divided
2 tablespoons cornstarch
1/2 cup (2 ounces) grated, reduced-fat cheese
3 tablespoons dry sherry (optional)
dash of paprika

Preheat oven to 350 degrees. Sprinkle fish fillets with butter-flavored sprinkles.

Roll up each fillet. Place seam side down in a covered baking dish that has been sprayed with nonstick cooking spray. Pour 1/4 cup milk over fillets. Cover and bake for 25 minutes, or until fish flakes easily.

Meanwhile, mix 1/2 cup milk with cornstarch and microwave on high for 50 seconds, stirring once halfway through cooking (or cook in saucepan, stirring constantly until thickened). Stir in cheese and sherry. Microwave for 20 seconds more (or continue to heat in saucepan).

Drain liquid from fish, discarding all but 1/2 cup. Add 1/2 cup of fish liquid to sauce. Pour over fish and sprinkle with paprika.

VARIATION: *Seafood-Stuffed Fillets*–Fill each fillet with a tablespoon of shrimp or crab before rolling up. Also add 1/2 cup shrimp or crab to the sauce.

This is a good recipe to serve for company. Adding shrimp or crab (see variation below) makes this a very special dish.

Makes 8 servings

Each Serving

Carb Servings
0

Exchanges
3 lean meat

Nutrient Analysis
calories 146
total fat 3g
saturated fat 1g
cholesterol 46mg
sodium 137mg
total carbohydrate 3g
dietary fiber 0g
sugars 1g
protein 26g

This recipe is a complete meal. It is very colorful and a good choice to serve when entertaining. Try tube-shaped or spiral pasta for variety.

Makes 7 1/2 cups
4 servings

Each Serving
1 3/4 cups

Carb Servings
2

Exchanges
1 1/2 starch
2 vegetable
2 lean meat

Nutrient Analysis
calories 249
total fat 2g
saturated fat 0g
cholesterol 37mg
sodium 245mg
total carbohydrate 32g
dietary fiber 5g
sugars 4g
protein 27g

Mediterranean Seafood

4 ounces uncooked pasta of your choice
8 ounces sliced mushrooms (about 3 cups)
2 red bell peppers, chopped (about 2 cups)
2 cups broccoli florets
1/2 cup sliced green onions
1 tablespoon chopped garlic
1 teaspoon Italian seasoning
1 teaspoon ground black pepper or lemon pepper
1/2 teaspoon salt (optional)
1 pound scallops or shelled and deveined shrimp
1/2 cup fat-free chicken broth*
grated Parmesan cheese (optional)

Cook pasta according to package directions. Drain and keep warm.

Meanwhile, spray a large skillet with nonstick cooking spray. Add seafood to skillet and cook until done. Remove from skillet and keep warm.

Add vegetables and seasonings to skillet. Stir-fry for about 4-5 minutes until crisp-tender. Add water or broth, as needed, to prevent sticking. Add seafood, brot,h and hot noodles to vegetables. Toss well. Cover and let set a couple of minutes before serving. If desired, top with Parmesan cheese.

NOTE: One serving is a good source of fiber.

*Sodium is figured for reduced sodium.

 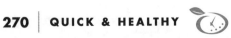

Shrimp Lettuce Wraps

1/4 cup rice vinegar
2 teaspoons sugar or the equivalent in artificial sweetener
1 pound cooked and cleaned salad shrimp
1/2 cup chopped green onion
1/4 cup chopped fresh cilantro
1/4 teaspoon crushed red pepper
1/4 teaspoon garlic powder
12 large lettuce leaves (bib or butter)

Optional Toppings:
mint leaves, chopped
dry-roasted peanuts, coarsely chopped

In a medium bowl, mix rice, vinegar, and sugar. Stir to dissolve. Add remaining ingredients, except the lettuce and optional toppings. If making in advance, add shrimp just before serving.

To serve, arrange bowl of shrimp, lettuce leaves, and optional toppings on serving area.

To make each lettuce wrap, place about 1/4 cup of shrimp mixture in a lettuce leaf. Add optional toppings. Roll up and enjoy!

This is a great warm weather dish. The optional toppings of peanuts and mint leaves add interest and flavor. Serve as an hors d'oeuvre or as a main dish. This also works well as a filling in pita bread halves.

Makes 12 wraps
4 servings

Each Serving
3 wraps

Carb Servings
0

Exchanges
3 lean meat

Nutrient Analysis
calories 129—with
   artificial sweetener 121
total fat 1g
saturated fat 0g
cholesterol 218mg
sodium 256mg
total carbohydrate 4g—
   with artificial sweetener
   2g
dietary fiber 1g
sugars 3g—with artificial
   sweetener 1g
protein 24g

Fresh cilantro and fresh ginger are especially good in this recipe. The chili paste is spicy-hot so use cautiously or omit if you don't like spicy foods.

Makes 5 cups
4 servings

Each Serving
1 1/4 cups

Carb Servings
1 1/2

Exchanges
1 fruit
1 vegetable
3 lean meat

Nutrient Analysis
calories 192—with
    artificial sweetener 179
total fat 1g
saturated fat 0g
cholesterol 37mg
sodium 588mg
total carbohydrate 24g—
    with artificial sweetener
    21g
dietary fiber 2g
sugars 14g—with artificial
    sweetener 11g
protein 22g

Spicy Seafood and Grapes

1 tablespoon cornstarch
3/4 cup fat-free chicken broth*, divided
2 tablespoons lite soy sauce
1 tablespoon granulated sugar or the equivalent in
    artificial sweetener
1 tablespoon red wine vinegar
1–2 teaspoons ground fresh chili paste** (optional)
1 pound scallops or shelled and deveined shrimp
3 tablespoons fresh minced ginger
1 tablespoon chopped garlic
2 cups broccoli florets
1 1/2 cups green seedless grapes
3/4 cup green onions, thinly sliced
1/4–1/2 cup fresh cilantro (optional)

In a small bowl, combine cornstarch and 1/4 cup chicken broth. Add soy sauce, sugar, vinegar, and chili paste.

Spray a skillet with nonstick cooking spray. Add seafood, ginger, and garlic. Stir-fry until seafood is cooked. Remove from skillet and keep warm.

Add broccoli to skillet and stir-fry until crisp tender, adding water or broth, as needed, to prevent sticking. Add grapes, green onions, and sauce mixture to the skillet. Bring to a boil, stirring constantly for 1–2 minutes or until thickened. Mix in cooked seafood. Top with cilantro just before serving.

Sodium is figured for reduced sodium.

**Found in the Asian section of the grocery store.*

Mandarin Orange Seafood

1 pound scallops or shelled and deveined shrimp
1 tablespoon minced fresh ginger
1–2 tablespoons lite soy sauce (optional)
1 cup green onions, sliced in 1-inch pieces
2 cups red bell pepper strips
1 tablespoon cornstarch
3/4 cup fat-free chicken broth*
1 can (11 ounces) mandarin oranges, in juice, drained
1 can (8 ounces) sliced water chestnuts, drained
hot cooked brown rice or noodles (optional)

Spray a large skillet with nonstick cooking spray. Add seafood, ginger, and soy sauce. Stir-fry a few minutes or until seafood is done. Remove from skillet and keep warm.

Add green onions and red pepper to skillet. Stir-fry until crisp tender, adding water or broth, as needed, to prevent sticking.

In a small bowl, mix cornstarch with chicken broth. Stir into skillet. Cook, stirring constantly, until thickened. Gently stir in cooked seafood, mandarin oranges, and water chestnuts. Heat thoroughly.

Serve over brown rice or noodles.

NOTE: One serving is a good source of fiber.

Sodium is figured for reduced sodium.

The addition of mandarin oranges gives a good flavor and eye appeal to the sauce. This colorful dish is one that you will want to serve for company.

Makes 4 cups
4 servings

Each Serving
1 cup

Carb Servings
1

Exchanges
1/2 fruit
2 vegetable
2 lean meat

Nutrient Analysis
calories 171
total fat 1g
saturated fat 0g
cholesterol 37mg
sodium 417mg
total carbohydrate 19g
dietary fiber 3g
sugars 7g
protein 21g

This recipe uses staple foods that I keep stocked in my cupboard. It's quick to put together and it has been one of my children's favorite dishes. Serve topped with Parmesan cheese.

Makes 5 cups
5 servings

Each Serving
1 cup

Carb Servings
2 1/2

Exchanges
2 1/2 starch
1 lean meat

Nutrient Analysis
calories 225
total fat 1g
saturated fat 0g
cholesterol 22mg
sodium 312mg
total carbohydrate 37g
dietary fiber 2g
sugars 2g
protein 16g

Clam Fettuccini

8 ounces uncooked fettuccini noodles (eggless)
3 cans (6.5 ounces each) minced clams, 2 drained and
　1 not drained
1 tablespoon chopped garlic
2 teaspoons lemon juice
1/2 teaspoon dried thyme

Cook noodles according to package directions. Drain.

Return noodles to pan and add remaining ingredients. Heat thoroughly. Turn off heat.

Cover and let set until liquid is absorbed, or if you prefer more moisture, serve immediately.

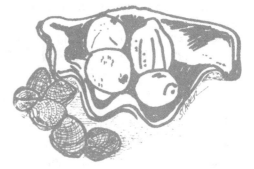

Lemon Basil Marinade

1/4 cup lemon juice
2 tablespoons olive oil
2 tablespoons finely chopped green onion
1/2 teaspoon dried basil or 1 tablespoon fresh
1/4 teaspoon salt (optional)

Mix all ingredients. Add fish and marinate for 1–4 hours in the refrigerator.

Drain marinade and broil or barbecue fish until done.

This amount is enough to marinate 1–2 pounds of seafood. The nutrition information is for the approximate amount of marinade retained in a cooked 3-ounce portion of seafood.

Makes 1/2 cup

Each Serving

Carb Servings
0

Exchanges
1/2 fat

Nutrient Analysis
calories 32
total fat 3g
saturated fat 0g
cholesterol 0mg
sodium 2mg
total carbohydrate 1g
dietary fiber 0g
sugars 0g
protein 0g

Soy Marinade

1/4 cup oil (canola or olive)
1/4 cup white wine
3 tablespoons lite soy sauce
2 tablespoons water
1 teaspoon chopped garlic
1/2 teaspoon ground ginger

Mix marinade ingredients. Add fish and marinate for 1–4 hours in the refrigerator.

Drain marinade and barbecue or broil fish until done.

This amount is enough to marinate 1–2 pounds of seafood. The nutrition information is for the approximate amount of marinade retained in a cooked 3-ounce portion of seafood.

Makes 3/4 cup

Each Serving

Carb Servings
0

Exchanges
1/2 fat

Nutrient Analysis
calories 24
total fat 2g
saturated fat 0g
cholesterol 0mg
sodium 72mg
total carbohydrate 0g
dietary fiber 0g
sugars 0g
protein 0g

Beef and Pork

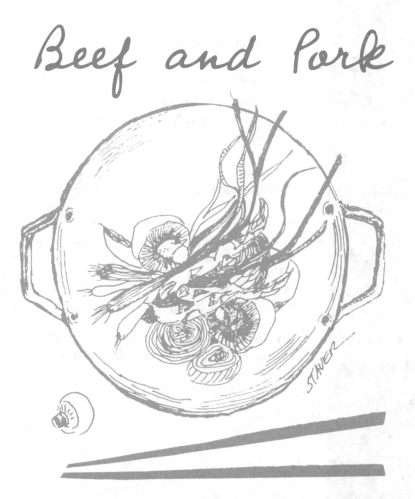

Lean beef and pork are good choices. Choose cuts such as top sirloin or tenderloin and trim off all visible fat. Less marbling also means less fat. Broiling or barbecuing are good methods for cooking since the fat drips out.

Breading and baking the pork chops makes the meat very moist and tender. You can find cornflake crumbs in the breadings section of the grocery store.

Makes 4 servings

Each Serving

Carb Servings
0

Exchanges
1/2 starch
3 lean meat

Nutrient Analysis
calories 167
total fat 5g
saturated fat 2g
cholesterol 62mg
sodium 91mg
total carbohydrate 5g
dietary fiber 0g
sugars 1g
protein 26g

Oven-Fried Pork Loin

1/4 cup cornflake crumbs
1/4 teaspoon dried thyme
1/4 teaspoon dried sage
1/8 teaspoon salt (optional)
1/8 teaspoon ground black pepper
1 pound boneless top loin pork chops (about 3/4-inch to 1-inch thick), well trimmed

Preheat oven to 350 degrees. Spray an 8-inch by 8-inch baking dish with nonstick cooking spray.

Mix the first five ingredients in a plastic bag. Place a couple pieces of pork in the plastic bag and shake to coat evenly.

Arrange pork in the baking pan so that they are not touching. Bake for 20–25 minutes or until pork is cooked.

VARIATION: *Italian Oven-Fried Pork*—Substitute 1/2 teaspoon of Italian seasoning for the sage and thyme.

Orange Pork Chops

1/3 cup sugar-free orange marmalade
2 tablespoons Dijon mustard
4 pork rib chops, with bone (cut 3 per pound)
3–4 bunches of green onions

In a small saucepan, mix marmalade and mustard. Stir over medium heat until marmalade is melted. Set aside.

Trim all fat from chops. Place chops on rack of a broiler pan or use the outdoor barbecue. Broil about 4 inches from the heat for 6 minutes. Turn chops and broil for 2 more minutes. Spoon half of the glaze over chops. Broil 4–5 minutes more or until chops are cooked.

Meanwhile, slice onions diagonally into 1-inch pieces. Spray a skillet with nonstick cooking spray. Add onions and stir-fry 2 minutes or until crisp-tender. Stir in remaining glaze and heat thoroughly. Serve over chops.

NOTE: One serving is a good source of fiber.

This is a delicious and unusual way to serve pork chops. It is a good dish for entertaining, especially if you use the outdoor barbecue.

Makes 4 servings

Each Serving

Carb Servings
1

Exchanges
1/2 carbohydrate
1 vegetable
3 lean meat

Nutrient Analysis
calories 223
total fat 8g
saturated fat 3g
cholesterol 62mg
sodium 246mg
total carbohydrate 13g
dietary fiber 3g
sugars 2g
protein 26g

Makes 4 cups
4 servings

Each Serving
1 cup

Carb Servings
2

Exchanges
1 1/2 starch
1 vegetable
3 lean meat

Nutrient Analysis
calories 297
total fat 7g
saturated fat 2g
cholesterol 66mg
sodium 381mg
total carbohydrate 30g
dietary fiber 3g
sugars 3g
protein 29g

Pork and Rice Casserole

1 cup uncooked quick-cooking brown rice
1 pound boneless pork top loin
1 cup chopped onion
1 cup sliced celery
1 can (10.75 ounces) low-fat condensed cream of
  celery soup*
1/2 can water
1/2 teaspoon dried marjoram
1/2 teaspoon dried thyme
1/4 teaspoon salt (optional)
1/4 teaspoon ground black pepper

Preheat oven to 350 degrees. Spray a covered 2-quart casserole with nonstick cooking spray. Spread rice in the casserole.

Cut pork into bite-size pieces. Brown pork in a skillet that has been sprayed with nonstick cooking spray. Top rice with pork, onion, and celery.

Mix seasonings and water with the soup. Pour over all. Cover and bake for 45 minutes. Let set 10 minutes before serving.

NOTE: One serving is a good source of fiber.

Sodium is figured for reduced sodium.

Chinese Pepper Steak

1 pound boneless beef top sirloin, cut into thin strips
2 cups fat-free beef broth*
2 green peppers, sliced
1 1/2 cups diagonally sliced celery
1 cup sliced onion
1 teaspoon chopped garlic
1/2 teaspoon salt (optional)
1/2 teaspoon ground black pepper
1/2 teaspoon sugar or the equivalent in artificial
   sweetener
1/4 cup cornstarch
2 teaspoons lite soy sauce
1/2 cup water

Spray a large skillet with nonstick cooking spray. Add beef
strips and stir-fry until browned. Add all but the last three
ingredients and simmer, covered, for 4–8 minutes.

Meanwhile, in a small bowl, mix cornstarch with soy
sauce and water. Stir into hot mixture and continue
cooking, stirring constantly, until thickened.

Serve over noodles or quick-cooking brown rice.

NOTE: One serving is a good source of fiber.

Sodium is figured for reduced sodium.

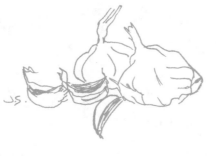

*This is a family favorite
that tastes great. If you
like crisp vegetables,
simmer for the lesser time.*

Makes 5 cups
4 servings

Each Serving
1 1/4 cups

Carb Servings
1

Exchanges
1/2 starch
2 vegetable
3 lean meat

Nutrient Analysis
calories 254—with
   artificial sweetener 252
total fat 9g
saturated fat 3g
cholesterol 66mg
sodium 388mg
total carbohydrate 16g
dietary fiber 3g
sugars 4g
protein 26g

Makes 5 cups
4 servings

Each Serving
1 1/4 cups

Carb Servings
1

Exchanges
1/2 starch
2 vegetable
3 lean meat

Nutrient Analysis
calories 219
total fat 5g
saturated fat 2g
cholesterol 62mg
sodium 366mg
total carbohydrate 16g
dietary fiber 2g
sugars 7g
protein 28g

Pork Chop Suey

1 pound boneless pork tenderloin
2 cups sliced celery
1 cup sliced onion
1 cup fat-free beef broth*
1 tablespoon lite soy sauce
1/4 teaspoon salt (optional)
2 1/2 tablespoons cornstarch
1/4 cup water
1 tablespoon molasses
1/4 teaspoon ground ginger
1 can (16 ounces) bean sprouts, drained and rinsed, or 1 pound fresh

Cut pork into 1-inch strips, about 1/4-inch thick. Brown pork in a large skillet that has been sprayed with nonstick cooking spray. Add the next five ingredients, cover, and simmer for 5–10 minutes.

Meanwhile, in a small bowl, mix cornstarch, water, molasses, and ginger. Stir into hot mixture and bring to a boil, stirring constantly until thickened.

Add bean sprouts and heat thoroughly. Serve over noodles or quick-cooking brown rice.

Sodium is figured for reduced sodium.

Beef or Pork Fajitas

1 pound boneless beef top sirloin or pork tenderloin
1 medium green bell pepper, sliced
1 medium onion, sliced
3 tablespoons lime juice
1/2 teaspoon dried coriander
1/2 teaspoon chili powder
4 (8-inch) or 8 (6-inch) whole-wheat tortillas
salsa (optional)

Cut meat into 1-inch strips. In a medium bowl, combine meat and vegetables.

Mix lime juice with coriander and chili powder. Pour over meat and vegetables. Set aside for a few minutes or for up to 1 hour.

Spray a skillet with nonstick cooking spray. Stir-fry meat and vegetables until done.

Warm tortillas in microwave about 50 seconds on high or in a nonstick skillet. Fill each tortilla with meat mixture. Serve with salsa.

NOTE: One serving is a good source of fiber.

This is a quick dish that the entire family will enjoy.

Makes 4 servings

Each Serving

Carb Servings
2

Exchanges
1 1/2 starch
2 vegetable
3 lean meat

Nutrient Analysis
calories 332
total fat 10g
saturated fat 3g
cholesterol 66mg
sodium 267mg
total carbohydrate 30g
dietary fiber 3g
sugars 6g
protein 29g

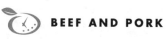

Makes 4 servings

Each Serving

Carb Servings
2

Exchanges
1 1/2 starch
1 vegetable
3 lean meat

Nutrient Analysis
calories 326
total fat 10g
saturated fat 3g
cholesterol 66mg
sodium 270mg
total carbohydrate 28g
dietary fiber 3g
sugars 5g
protein 29g

Fajitas Barbecue Style

Marinade:
1/3 cup lime juice
1 teaspoon dried oregano
1 teaspoon chili powder
1/2 teaspoon garlic powder
1/4 teaspoon salt (optional)
1/4 teaspoon ground black pepper

1 pound boneless beef top sirloin steak, 1-inch thick
4 (8-inch) or 8 (6-inch) whole-wheat tortillas
1 cup each: shredded lettuce and chopped tomato
1/2 cup sliced green onion

Mix marinade ingredients in a container large enough to hold the steak. Add steak, coating both sides with the marinade. Refrigerate for 1 hour, turning halfway through marinating time. Drain marinade and discard.

Broil or barbecue steak about 2–3 minutes on each side or until desired doneness. Carve cross grain into thin slices.

Heat tortillas in microwave or in a nonstick skillet. To serve, portion meat, lettuce, tomato, and onions on tortillas.

NOTE: One serving is a good source of fiber.

Marinated Steak

Marinade:
1/3 cup lite soy sauce
1/3 cup chili sauce
1/4 cup water
1 tablespoon Worcestershire sauce
1 tablespoon dried parsley
1 teaspoon dried oregano
1/4 teaspoon ground black pepper
1/4 teaspoon garlic powder
1/8 teaspoon chili powder
1/8 teaspoon ground mustard

1 1/2 pounds boneless steak (top sirloin, flank, or round), well trimmed

Mix marinade ingredients in a container large enough to hold the steak.

Add steak, coating both sides with the marinade. Refrigerate and marinate for 2–4 hours, turning steak once halfway through the marinating time. Drain and discard marinade.

Broil or barbecue steak about 2–3 minutes on each side or until desired doneness. Carve cross grain into thin slices.

This is a favorite marinade for steaks. It really adds a good flavor.

Makes 6 servings

Each Serving

Carb Servings
0

Exchanges
3 lean meat

Nutrient Analysis
calories 183
total fat 9g
saturated fat 3g
cholesterol 66mg
sodium 396mg
total carbohydrate 1g
dietary fiber 0g
sugars 0g
protein 24g

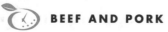

Makes 4 servings

Each Serving

Carb Servings
1/2

Exchanges
2 vegetable
3 lean meat

Nutrient Analysis
calories 213
total fat 9g
saturated fat 3g
cholesterol 66mg
sodium 145mg
total carbohydrate 8g
dietary fiber 3g
sugars 4g
protein 25g

Beef or Pork Stir-Fry

1 pound boneless top sirloin beef or pork top loin
1 teaspoon chopped garlic
2 cups fresh broccoli florets
1 cup sliced carrots
1 cup sliced red bell pepper
1 small zucchini, cut into strips
1–2 teaspoons lite soy sauce
1/4 teaspoon ground black pepper

Cut meat into strips 1/4-inch thick.

Spray a skillet with nonstick cooking spray. Add meat and stir-fry with garlic until browned. Remove and keep warm.

Stir-fry carrots until partially done. Add water or broth, as needed, to prevent sticking. Add remaining vegetables and stir-fry a few minutes. Add meat, soy sauce, and pepper. Continue to stir-fry until vegetables and meat are done to your liking.

Serve with rice or noodles.

Cooking tip: Vegetables that also work well in this recipe are green, yellow, or orange bell peppers; baby corn; celery; green, red, or yellow onions; cauliflower; cabbage; snow peas; mushrooms; and bean sprouts.

NOTE: One serving is a good source of fiber.

VARIATION: *Chicken Stir-Fry*–Substitute skinless, boneless chicken breasts for the meat.

Ground Meat Dishes

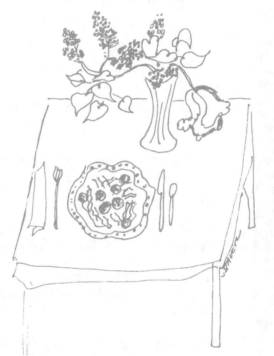

Ground beef, ground turkey, or ground venison or elk may be used in any of the recipes in this section. When buying ground beef or turkey, look for 7% fat or less. If you have wild meat butchered, ask not to have fat added to the meat.

Makes 12 wraps
4 servings

Each Serving
3 wraps

Carb Servings
0

Exchanges
1 vegetable
3 lean meat

Nutrient Analysis
calories 177
total fat 8g
saturated fat 3g
cholesterol 70mg
sodium 108mg
total carbohydrate 4g
dietary fiber 1g
sugars 2g
protein 23g

Beef Lettuce Wraps

1 pound extra-lean ground beef or ground turkey (7% fat)
1/2 cup sliced green onion
2 tablespoons minced fresh ginger
2 tablespoons orange juice
2 tablespoons lime juice
1/2–1 teaspoon ground fresh chili paste*
1/4 teaspoon salt (optional)
1/2 cup chopped fresh cilantro
12 large lettuce leaves (bib or butter)

Optional Toppings:
mint leaves, chopped
dry-roasted peanuts, coarsely chopped

In a medium saucepan that has been sprayed with
nonstick cooking spray, sauté meat with onion and ginger.
Add orange juice, lime juice, chili paste, and salt. Simmer
about 10 minutes or until meat is cooked. Add cilantro.

To serve: Arrange bowl of meat mixture, lettuce leaves,
and optional toppings on serving area.

To make each lettuce wrap, place about 1/4 cup of meat
mixture in a lettuce leaf. Add optional toppings. Roll up
and enjoy!

*Found in the Asian section of the grocery store. It is spicy-hot so use
sparingly or omit if you don't like spicy foods.*

Turkey Lettuce Wraps

1 pound extra-lean ground turkey (7% fat)
1/2 cup sliced green onion
2 tablespoons minced fresh ginger
1 can (8 ounces) sliced water chestnuts, drained and chopped
1 teaspoon sesame oil
1 teaspoon lite soy sauce
1/4 teaspoon salt (optional)
1/4 cup chopped fresh cilantro
12 large lettuce leaves (bib or butter)

Optional Toppings:
mint leaves, chopped
dry-roasted peanuts, coarsely chopped

In a medium saucepan that has been sprayed with nonstick cooking spray, sauté turkey with onion and ginger. Add water chestnuts, oil, soy sauce, and salt.

Continue to cook until meat is done. Add cilantro. To serve, arrange bowl of meat mixture, lettuce leaves, and optional toppings on serving area.

To make each lettuce wrap, place about 1/4 cup of meat mixture in a lettuce leaf. Add optional toppings. Roll up and enjoy!

This Asian dish can be served wrapped in lettuce or in pita bread. Serve as an hors d'oeuvre, sandwich, or a main dish. The turkey provides a mild flavor and the chestnuts add a crunchy texture.

Makes 12 wraps
4 servings

Each Serving
3 wraps

Carb Servings
1/2

Exchanges
1 vegetable
3 lean meat

Nutrient Analysis
calories 192
total fat 8g
saturated fat 2g
cholesterol 48mg
sodium 137mg
total carbohydrate 7g
dietary fiber 2g
sugars 1g
protein 23g

These patties are so moist and have such a good flavor. You can also shape into a meatloaf instead of patties. I prefer using oat bran, as it blends in better.

Makes 4 servings
4 patties

Each Serving
1 patty

Carb Servings
1/2

Exchanges
1/2 starch
3 lean meat

Nutrient Analysis
calories 222
total fat 9g
saturated fat 3g
cholesterol 71mg
sodium 127mg
total carbohydrate 9g
dietary fiber 1g
sugars 2g
protein 26g

Meat Patties

1/2 cup oatmeal or oat bran
1/2 cup fat-free milk
1/4 cup egg substitute (equal to 1 egg)
1/2 tablespoon dried parsley
1 teaspoon ground mustard
1 teaspoon dried or 1 tablespoon fresh minced onion
1/2 teaspoon salt (optional)
1/4 teaspoon chopped garlic
1/4 teaspoon ground black pepper
1 pound extra-lean ground beef or ground turkey (7% fat)

Mix the first nine ingredients. Add ground meat and mix well. Shape into four patties. Cook in the microwave, in the conventional oven, or on the barbecue.

CONVENTIONAL OVEN: Preheat oven to 425 degrees. Arrange patties on a baking pan that has been sprayed with nonstick cooking spray. Bake for 20 minutes.

MICROWAVE OVEN: Arrange meat patties in a circle, on a microwave-safe dish, leaving the center empty. Cover with wax paper and cook on high for 7–8 minutes, rotating 1/4 turn halfway through cooking time.

BARBECUE: Cook over hot coals, turning once, until done.

Baked Meatballs

1 cup oatmeal or oat bran
1 cup fat-free milk
1/2 cup egg substitute (equal to 2 eggs)
1 tablespoon dried parsley
2 teaspoons onion powder
1 teaspoon salt (optional)
1/2 teaspoon ground black pepper
1/4 teaspoon ground nutmeg
2 pounds extra-lean ground beef or ground turkey (7% fat)

Preheat oven to 425 degrees.

Mix the first eight ingredients. Add ground meat and mix well. Shape into 1 1/2-inch balls.

Arrange on baking sheets that have been sprayed with nonstick cooking spray. Bake for 12 minutes or until done.

Baked Meatballs are used in the following recipes:
Swedish Meatballs, page 293
Spaghetti and Meatballs, page 292
Meatball Sandwich, page 196

These are so quick because you cook them in the oven. Make this large amount and freeze for later use in the recipes listed.

Makes 48 meatballs
12 servings

Each Serving
4 meatballs

Carb Servings
1/2

Exchanges
1/2 starch
2 lean meat

Nutrient Analysis
calories 146
total fat 6g
saturated fat 2g
cholesterol 47mg
sodium 85mg
total carbohydrate 6g
dietary fiber 1g
sugars 1g
protein 17g

This is an easy recipe if you have meatballs in the freezer and sauce in the cupboard. Complete the meal with a tossed salad.

Makes 6 servings
4 meatballs with sauce
   and 1/2 cup noodles

Each Serving

Carb Servings
2

Exchanges
2 starch
2 lean meat
1/2 fat

Nutrient Analysis
calories 277
total fat 9g
saturated fat 2g
cholesterol 47mg
sodium 591mg
total carbohydrate 28g
dietary fiber 4g
sugars 8g
protein 21g

Spaghetti and Meatballs

24 Baked Meatballs (page 291)
1 jar (26 ounces) spaghetti sauce (less than 4 grams fat per 4 ounces)
3 cups cooked spaghetti noodles (3 1/2 ounces dry)

Heat meatballs in sauce. Serve over spaghetti noodles.

NOTE: One serving is a good source of fiber.

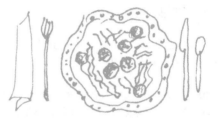

Swedish Meatballs

20 Baked Meatballs (page 291)
1 can (14.5 ounces) fat-free beef or chicken broth*
3 1/2 tablespoons unbleached all-purpose flour

Pour 1/4 of the broth in a covered container. Add flour and shake well to prevent lumps.

In a saucepan, combine remainder of broth with the flour mixture. Bring to a boil, stirring constantly with a wire whisk, until thickened. Add meatballs and heat.

VARIATION: *Swedish Meatballs and Mushrooms*—Add one small can of mushrooms, drained and rinsed, to the gravy when adding the meatballs.

Cooking tip: This is quick to prepare if you have meatballs in the freezer and sauce in the cupboard.

Sodium is figured for reduced sodium.

This is a family favorite. It tastes great over mashed potatoes, rice, or noodles.

Makes 4 servings

Each Serving
5 meatballs plus 1/2 cup sauce

Carb Servings
1

Exchanges
1 starch
3 lean meat

Nutrient Analysis
calories 214
total fat 8g
saturated fat 3g
cholesterol 59mg
sodium 264mg
total carbohydrate 13g
dietary fiber 2g
sugars 1g
protein 23g

The canned soup in this recipe makes a nice gravy. Bite-size broccoli pieces can be substituted for the asparagus. When preparing asparagus, snap off the fibrous end and soak the tips in water to remove any dirt.

Makes 4 servings

Each Serving

Carb Servings
1

Exchanges
1 starch
1 vegetable
3 lean meat

Nutrient Analysis
calories 286
total fat 10g
saturated fat 4g
cholesterol 73mg
sodium 469mg
total carbohydrate 19g
dietary fiber 4g
sugars 4g
protein 29g

Asparagus-Topped Meatloaf

1/2 cup oatmeal or oat bran
1/4 cup fat-free milk
1/4 cup egg substitute (equal to 1 egg)
1/2 tablespoon dried parsley
1/2 teaspoon salt (optional)
1/4 teaspoon ground black pepper
1 pound extra-lean ground beef or ground turkey (7% fat)
3/4 pound asparagus spears, trimmed, or 3 cups bite-size broccoli florets
1 can (13 ounces) mushroom pieces and stems, drained and rinsed
1 can (10.75 ounces) low-fat, condensed cream of mushroom soup*
1/4 can water
1/2 teaspoon paprika
1/8 teaspoon ground black pepper

Preheat oven to 350 degrees. Combine the first six ingredients. Add ground meat and mix well. Press meat mixture in an 8-inch by 8-inch baking pan that has been sprayed with nonstick cooking spray.

If asparagus spears are very thick, cut in half, lengthwise. Arrange vegetables over meat.

Mix soup and water. Spread over vegetables. Sprinkle with paprika and pepper. Bake for 40 minutes or until asparagus is crisp-tender and meat is cooked.

NOTE: One serving is a good source of fiber.

Sodium is figured for reduced sodium.

 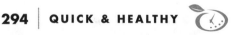

Pizza Meat Loaf

1 pound extra-lean ground beef or ground turkey (7% fat)
1/4 cup pizza sauce
1 cup thin sliced vegetables such as green pepper
  and onion
1/4 cup (1 ounce) grated, reduced-fat mozzarella cheese
  (optional)

Spray a 9-inch glass pie plate with nonstick cooking spray. Pack the meat lightly onto the pie plate. Follow the directions below for microwave or conventional oven.

CONVENTIONAL OVEN: Preheat oven to 425 degrees. Bake for 12–14 minutes. Drain any liquid. Top with pizza sauce, vegetables, and cheese (optional). Return to oven for 5 minutes.

MICROWAVE OVEN: Cover with wax paper and cook on high for 6 minutes, turning 1/4 turn halfway through cooking time. Drain any liquid. Top with pizza sauce, vegetables, and cheese (optional). Cook on high for about 1–2 minutes.

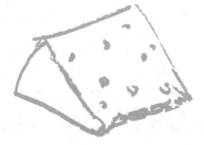

This is a family favorite that can be put together in a hurry. Serve with a salad and a whole-grain roll.

Makes 4 servings

Each Serving

Carb Servings
0

Exchanges
3 lean meat

Nutrient Analysis
calories 172
total fat 8g
saturated fat 3g
cholesterol 70mg
sodium 151mg
total carbohydrate 2g
dietary fiber 1g
sugars 1g
protein 22g

The vegetables add a good flavor to this meat loaf. Use the microwave method and have it ready in less than 30 minutes.

Makes 6 servings

Each Serving

Carb Servings
1

Exchanges
1/2 starch
1 vegetable
3 lean meat

Nutrient Analysis
calories 244
total fat 9g
saturated fat 3g
cholesterol 71mg
sodium 341mg
total carbohydrate 16g
dietary fiber 2g
sugars 7g
protein 26g

Meat Loaf

3/4 cup oatmeal or oat bran
3/4 cup fat-free milk
1/2 cup catsup
1/4 cup egg substitute (equal to 1 egg)
1 tablespoon dried parsley
1 teaspoon ground mustard
1 teaspoon salt (optional)
1/2 teaspoon chopped garlic
1/2 teaspoon ground black pepper
1/2 cup finely chopped onion
1/2 cup finely chopped green pepper or celery
1 1/2 pounds extra-lean ground beef or ground turkey (7% fat)

Mix the first nine ingredients. Add vegetables and ground meat. Mix well. Follow the directions below for microwave or conventional oven.

CONVENTIONAL OVEN: Preheat oven to 325 degrees. Pack meat mixture in a loaf pan that has been sprayed with nonstick cooking spray. Bake for 1 hour.

MICROWAVE OVEN: Pack meat mixture lightly into a 10-inch glass dish that has been sprayed with nonstick cooking spray, making a well in the center. Place empty glass, right side down, in center of dish. Cover with wax paper and cook on high for 18 minutes, rotating 1/4 turn after 6 minutes and again after another 6 minutes of cooking time. Let rest for 5 minutes before serving.

Quick Meat Lasagna

1 pound extra-lean ground beef or ground turkey (7% fat)
1 teaspoon chopped garlic
3/4 teaspoon anise seed
1/2 teaspoon fennel seed
2 cups low-fat cottage cheese or Ricotta cheese
2 tablespoons dried parsley
4 cups spaghetti sauce (less than 4 g fat per 4 ounces)*
3/4 pound uncooked lasagna noodles (12 noodles)
1 cup (4 ounces) grated, reduced-fat mozzarella cheese
1/4 cup grated Parmesan cheese

Preheat oven to 350 degrees. Brown meat and garlic with anise and fennel in a skillet that has been sprayed with nonstick cooking spray. Cook until done.

Mix cottage cheese, ground meat, and parsley.

Spray a 9-inch by 13-inch baking pan with nonstick cooking spray. Pour 1 cup of sauce in bottom of pan. Layer in this order: 4 noodles, 1/2 meat mixture, 1/2 mozzarella, 1 cup sauce, 4 noodles, 1/2 meat mixture, 1/2 mozzarella, 1 cup sauce, 4 noodles, and the rest of the sauce. Sprinkle with Parmesan cheese.

Bake, covered tightly with aluminum foil, for 1 hour. Increase baking time by 15 minutes if it has been refrigerated.

Or one jar (1 pound, 10 ounces) and water to equal 4 cups.

You don't precook the noodles in this recipe, so it is really fast to assemble. This can be put together the night before and refrigerated without baking.

Makes 12 servings

Each Serving

Carb Servings
2

Exchanges
2 starch
2 lean meat

Nutrient Analysis
calories 265
total fat 7g
saturated fat 3g
cholesterol 31mg
sodium 595mg
total carbohydrate 29g
dietary fiber 2g
sugars 7g
protein 21g

Vegetables and smoked sausage go together to make a delicious and healthy dish. The addition of the barbecue sauce adds a good flavor.

Makes 6 cups
5 servings

Each Serving
about 1 cup

Carb Servings
1

Exchanges
1/2 starch
2 vegetable
2 lean meat

Nutrient Analysis
calories 203
total fat 8g
saturated fat 3g
cholesterol 56mg
sodium 1013mg
total carbohydrate 17g
dietary fiber 3g
sugars 12g
protein 15g

Barbecued Smoked Sausage and Cabbage Casserole

4 cups chopped cabbage (about 12 ounces)
1 cup chopped onion
1 cup sliced celery
1 cup sliced bell pepper, red or green
1 package (16 ounces) low-fat turkey smoked sausage, cut into slices
1/3 cup barbecue sauce

Preheat oven to 350 degrees.

In a large bowl, combine all ingredients and mix well.

Spray a 2 1/2-quart covered casserole with nonstick cooking spray. Add all ingredients. Cover and bake for 30–40 minutes.

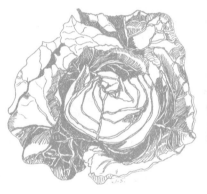

NOTE: One serving is a good source of fiber.

This recipe is higher in sodium and should be limited by those on a low-sodium diet.

VARIATION: *Smoked Sausage and Creamy Vegetables*– Substitute 1 can (10.75 ounces) low-fat, condensed cream of celery soup for the barbecue sauce. This makes a nice creamy sauce.

 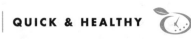

Sausage and Sauerkraut

1 jar (32 ounces) sauerkraut
2 cups unpeeled new potatoes, thinly sliced
1/2 cup onion, thinly sliced
1 pound low-fat turkey smoked sausage, cut into 10 pieces

Drain sauerkraut. Add water and drain. Add water and drain again.

Follow the directions below for microwave or conventional oven.

CONVENTIONAL OVEN: Preheat oven to 350 degrees. Place sauerkraut in a 2-quart covered casserole that has been sprayed with nonstick cooking spray. Top with potatoes, onions, and sausage. Cover and cook for 1 hour or until potatoes are tender.

MICROWAVE OVEN: Add potatoes and onions to a 2-quart glass-covered casserole. Cover and cook on high for 5 minutes, stirring once halfway through cooking time. Top potatoes with sauerkraut and sausage. Cover and microwave on high for 7 minutes, stirring halfway through cooking time.

NOTE: One serving is an excellent source of fiber.

This recipe is higher in sodium and should be limited by those on a low-sodium diet.

VARIATION: *Sausage and Cabbage*—Substitute shredded cabbage for all or part of the sauerkraut. Cook with potatoes, before adding sausage, when using the microwave.

*Half of the grams of fiber have been subtracted from the grams of total carbohydrate when figuring Carb Servings.

The sodium from the sauerkraut is significantly reduced by rinsing it twice, however, it can be reduced further by substituting cabbage.

Makes 8 cups
5 servings

Each Serving
about 1 1/2 cups

Carb Servings*
1

Exchanges
1 starch
1 vegetable
2 lean meat

Nutrient Analysis
calories 230
total fat 8g
saturated fat 3g
cholesterol 56mg
sodium 1272mg
total carbohydrate 22g
dietary fiber 6g
sugars 7g
protein 15g

This is another complete meal that will be a family pleaser. If you like cabbage more crisp, cook for the lesser amount of time. Ground turkey works best in this recipe.

Makes 8 cups
4 servings

Each Serving
2 cups

Carb Servings
2 1/2

Exchanges
1 1/2 starch
3 vegetable
3 lean meat

Nutrient Analysis
calories 345
total fat 9g
saturated fat 2g
cholesterol 68mg
sodium 398mg
total carbohydrate 39g
dietary fiber 5g
sugars 8g
protein 28g

Creamy Cabbage Stir-Fry

4 ounces uncooked egg noodles (eggless)
    (about 3 cups dry)
1 pound extra-lean ground turkey or beef (7% fat)
1 1/2 cups chopped onion
1/2 teaspoon salt (optional)
1/4 teaspoon ground black pepper
1 can (10.75 ounces) low-fat condensed cream of
    celery soup*
4 cups chopped cabbage (about 10 ounces)

Cook noodles according to package directions. Drain.

Spray a large skillet with nonstick cooking spray. Brown ground meat with onion and seasonings. Add cream soup and mix well. Add cabbage and reduce heat to low.

Cover and cook for 10–15 minutes or until cabbage is cooked to your liking. Add cooked noodles and mix well.

NOTE: One serving is an excellent source of fiber.

Sodium is figured for reduced sodium.

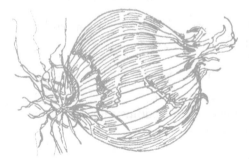

Tortilla Pie

2 pounds extra-lean ground beef or ground turkey (7% fat)

2 large onions, chopped

2 cups thick and chunky salsa

1 can (8 ounces) tomato sauce*

1 teaspoon each: ground cumin, chili powder, and garlic powder

1 can (15 ounces) creamed corn

12 corn tortillas (6-inch), cut into 1-inch strips

3/4 cup (3 ounces) grated, reduced-fat cheddar cheese or Mexican blend cheese

Preheat oven to 350 degrees.

Spray a large skillet with nonstick cooking spray. Add ground meat and onion and cook until done. Remove from heat. Add salsa, sauce, seasonings, and corn. Mix well.

Spray a 9-inch by 13-inch baking pan with nonstick cooking spray.

Layer mixture with the tortillas, starting with 1/4 of the meat mixture and topping with 1/3 of the tortilla strips. Continue layering, ending with the meat mixture. Cover and bake for 35–40 minutes or until thoroughly heated. Add cheese and cook another 5 minutes.

NOTE: One serving is a good source of fiber.

Sodium is figured for no added salt.

This makes a large amount, so serve this for company or plan on having leftovers. Children really like this recipe.

Makes 10 servings

Each Serving

Carb Servings
2

Exchanges
1 1/2 starch
2 vegetable
3 lean meat

Nutrient Analysis
calories 288
total fat 9g
saturated fat 3g
cholesterol 62mg
sodium 533mg
total carbohydrate 31g
dietary fiber 3g
sugars 6g
protein 23g

Makes 7 cups
6 servings

Each Serving
about 1 cup

Carb Servings
2

Exchanges
1 starch
2 vegetable
3 lean meat

Nutrient Analysis
calories 290
total fat 8g
saturated fat 3g
cholesterol 56mg
sodium 248mg
total carbohydrate 31g
dietary fiber 3g
sugars 7g
protein 24g

John Torrey

6 ounces uncooked elbow macaroni
1 pound extra-lean ground beef or ground turkey (7% fat)
1/2 green pepper, chopped
1 small onion, chopped
1 can (14.5 ounces) diced tomatoes*
1 can (8 ounces) tomato sauce*
1 can (4 ounces) mushroom pieces and stems, drained and rinsed
3/4 cup (3 ounces) grated, reduced-fat cheddar cheese
1/2 teaspoon chopped garlic
1/2 teaspoon chili powder
1/4 teaspoon salt (optional)

Preheat oven to 350 degrees. Cook macaroni according to package directions. Drain.

Spray a large skillet with nonstick cooking spray. Add ground meat, green pepper, and onion. Sauté until meat is cooked. Add remaining ingredients and macaroni. Pour into a 2 1/2-quart covered casserole that has been sprayed with nonstick cooking spray.

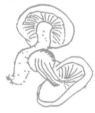

Bake, covered, for 35–40 minutes or until thoroughly heated.

NOTE: One serving is a good source of fiber.

Sodium is figured for no added salt.

Moore

6 ounces uncooked fettuccini noodles (eggless)
1 pound extra-lean ground beef or ground turkey (7% fat)
1 can (10.75 ounces) condensed tomato soup*
1/8 teaspoon ground black pepper
1/4 cup (1 ounce) grated, reduced-fat cheddar cheese
  (optional)

Cook fettuccini according to package directions. Drain.

Brown meat in a skillet that has been sprayed with
nonstick cooking spray. Add soup, pepper, and cooked
fettuccini. Cook over low heat until hot.

Optional: Top with cheese and cover for a couple of
minutes or until cheese is melted.

Sodium is figured for reduced sodium.

*This is another quick dish
that your family will enjoy.*

Makes 5 cups
4 servings

Each Serving
1 1/4 cups

Carb Servings
3

Exchanges
2 starch
2 vegetable
3 lean meat

Nutrient Analysis
calories 374
total fat 10g
saturated fat 3g
cholesterol 70mg
sodium 379mg
total carbohydrate 41g
dietary fiber 2g
sugars 8g
protein 29g

Makes 4 cups
4 servings

Each Serving
1 cup

Carb Servings*
1 1/2

Exchanges*
1 1/2 starch
3 lean meat

Nutrient Analysis
calories 293
total fat 8g
saturated fat 3g
cholester 70mg
sodium 692mg
total carbohydrate 26g
dietary fiber 6g
sugars 7g
protein 28g

Quick Meat and Bean Supper

1 pound extra-lean ground beef or ground turkey (7% fat)
1/2 cup chopped onion
1 can (15 ounces) fat-free vegetarian baked beans
3 tablespoons catsup

Spray a skillet with nonstick cooking spray. Brown ground meat with onion and cook until done.

Add remaining ingredients and heat thoroughly.

NOTE: One serving is an excellent source of fiber.

This recipe is higher in sodium and should be limited by those on a low-sodium diet.

Half of the grams of fiber have been subtracted from the grams of total carbohydrate when figuring Carb Servings and Exchanges.

Biscuits and Gravy

1 can (7 ounces) buttermilk biscuits* (10 biscuits per can)
1 package (2.6 ounces) country gravy**
1 pound extra-lean ground beef or ground turkey (7% fat)

Prepare the biscuits and country gravy following the package directions.

Meanwhile, cook ground meat in a skillet that has been sprayed with nonstick cooking spray.

When the gravy is thickened, mix with the cooked meat. To serve, split biscuits and top with gravy.

This recipe is higher in sodium and should be limited by those on a low-sodium diet.

*Look for biscuits that are only 100 calories, 1.5 grams of fat, and 1 gram of fiber for 2 biscuits.

**Look for country gravy with no more than 2 grams of fat per serving and no saturated or trans fats.*

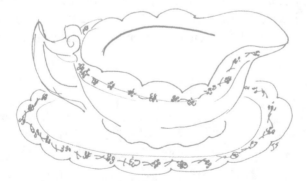

We were able to make a low-fat version of this popular dish.

Makes 5 servings

Each Serving
2 biscuits and 2/3 cup gravy

Carb Servings
2

Exchanges
2 starch
2 lean meat
1 fat

Nutrient Analysis
calories 292
total fat 11g
saturated fat 3g
cholesterol 63mg
sodium 876mg
total carbohydrate 28g
dietary fiber 1g
sugars 6g
protein 22g

Makes 6 servings

Each Serving

Carb Servings
1/2

Exchanges
1/2 fat-free milk
2 lean meat

Nutrient Analysis
calories 120
total fat 3g
saturated fat 1g
cholesterol 27mg
sodium 219mg
total carbohydrate 6g
dietary fiber 0g
sugars 4g
protein 17g

Crustless Quiche with Ground Meat

1/2 pound extra-lean ground beef or ground turkey (7% fat)
1/4 teaspoon salt (optional)
1/8 teaspoon ground black pepper
1 1/2 cups egg substitute (equal to 6 eggs)
1/2 cup fat-free sour cream
1/2 cup fat-free plain yogurt or 1/2 cup fat-free milk
1/3 cup sliced green onion
1/4 cup (1 ounce) grated, reduced-fat cheddar cheese

Preheat oven to 350 degrees. Brown ground meat, with seasonings, in a skillet that has been sprayed with nonstick cooking spray.

In a medium bowl, using a wire whisk, beat eggs with sour cream and yogurt (or milk) until smooth. Mix in onion and ground meat.

Spray a 9-inch pie pan with nonstick cooking spray. Pour egg mixture into pan. Bake for 35 minutes or until a knife inserted in the center comes out clean. Top with cheese and return to oven for 2 minutes or until cheese is melted.

Desserts

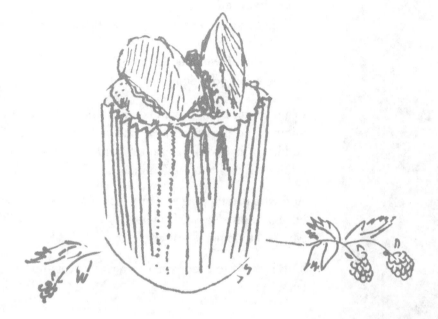

Some of the quick-to-prepare desserts in this section use sugar-free gelatin or sugar-free pudding. Many can be prepared in as little as 10 minutes. All of the recipes in this section are lower in sugar and fat than most desserts.

So good and so quick! This impressive dessert can be prepared just a few minutes before company arrives.

Makes 6 cups
8 servings

Each Serving
3/4 cup

Carb Servings
1

Exchanges
1 1/2 carbohydrate

Nutrient Analysis
calories 104
total fat 0g
saturated fat 0g
cholesterol 2mg
sodium 279mg
total carbohydrate 20g
dietary fiber 1g
sugars 8g
protein 3g

Chocolate Mocha Mousse

3 cups fat-free milk
1 tablespoon instant coffee crystals, regular or decaffeinated
1 large box (2.1 ounces) sugar-free instant chocolate pudding
3 cups fat-free whipped topping (8-ounce container)
fat-free whipped topping (optional)

In a medium bowl, mix milk with coffee. Let set a few minutes and then stir until coffee is dissolved. Add pudding mix and stir constantly with a wire whisk for 2 minutes. Refrigerate for 5 minutes.

Add whipped topping and mix well. Pour into a serving bowl or individual parfait glasses. Garnish with additional whipped topping, if desired.

This is ready to eat or you can refrigerate it and serve later.

Coffee Mousse

3 cups fat-free milk
2 tablespoons instant coffee crystals, regular or
  decaffeinated
1 large box (1.5 ounces) sugar-free instant vanilla pudding
3 cups fat-free whipped topping (8-ounce container)
fat-free whipped topping (optional)

In a medium bowl, mix milk with coffee. Let set a few
minutes and then stir until coffee is dissolved. Add
pudding mix and stir constantly with a wire whisk for 2
minutes. Refrigerate for 5 minutes.

Add whipped topping and mix
well. Pour into a serving bowl
or individual parfait glasses.

Garnish with additional
whipped topping, if desired.
This is ready to eat or you can
refrigerate it and serve later.

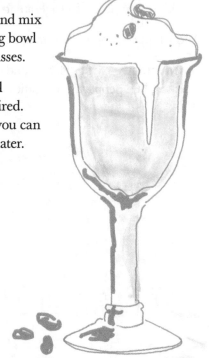

*A must for coffee lovers.
This light dessert can
also be served over angel
food cake.*

Makes 6 cups
8 servings

Each Serving
3/4 cup

Carb Servings
1

Exchanges
1 carbohydrate

Nutrient Analysis
calories 98
total fat 0g
saturated fat 0g
cholesterol 2mg
sodium 301mg
total carbohydrate 19g
dietary fiber 0g
sugars 8g
protein 3g

Makes 4 cups
5 servings

Each Serving
about 3/4 cup

Carb Servings
1

Exchanges
1 carbohydrate

Nutrient Analysis
calories 102
total fat 0g
saturated fat 0g
cholesterol 2mg
sodium 313mg
total carbohydrate 19g
dietary fiber 0g
sugars 8g
protein 3g

Peppermint Mousse

1 small box (1 ounce) sugar-free instant white chocolate
  pudding
2 cups fat-free milk
1/2 teaspoon peppermint extract
3–4 drops red food coloring
2 cups fat-free whipped topping
5 crushed peppermint candies (optional), regular or
  sugar-free

In a medium bowl, mix pudding with milk, peppermint
extract, and food coloring. Stir constantly with a wire
whisk for 2 minutes. Refrigerate for 5 minutes.

Add whipped topping and mix well.

Spoon into five parfait glasses and serve as is or topped
with crushed peppermint candies or a candy cane.

White Chocolate Mousse with Berries

1 small box (1 ounce) sugar-free instant white chocolate pudding
2 cups fat-free milk
2 cups fat-free whipped topping
2 cups fresh berries (or frozen, thawed) such as raspberries, blueberries, or huckleberries

In a medium bowl, mix pudding with milk. Stir constantly with a wire whisk for 2 minutes. Refrigerate for 5 minutes.

Add whipped topping and mix well. Layer mousse with berries in a serving bowl or individual parfait glasses. Be sure to save some berries for the top.

This is ready to eat or you can refrigerate it and serve later.

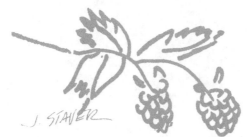

J. STAVER

Try this very light and refreshing dessert. It is so quick to prepare! Use a variety of berries alone or in combination. When fresh berries are not available, substitute frozen berries that have been thawed.

Makes 6 cups
8 servings

Each Serving
3/4 cup

Carb Servings
1

Exchanges
1 carbohydrate

Nutrient Analysis
calories 78
total fat 0g
saturated fat 0g
cholesterol 1mg
sodium 196mg
total carbohydrate 16g
dietary fiber 2g
sugars 6g
protein 2g

This is a refreshing dessert that takes just minutes to prepare. It looks especially good served in individual parfait glasses.

Makes 4 cups
5 servings

Each Serving
3/4 cup

Carb Servings
1 1/2

Exchanges
1 1/2 carbohydrate

Nutrient Analysis
calories 115
total fat 0g
saturated fat 0g
cholesterol 2mg
sodium 332mg
total carbohydrate 22g
dietary fiber 0g
sugars 9g
protein 3g

Grasshopper Mousse

1 small box (1 ounce) sugar-free instant white chocolate pudding
2 cups fat-free milk
1/2 teaspoon peppermint extract
3–4 drops green food coloring
2 cups fat-free whipped topping
2 chocolate graham cracker squares, crushed

In a medium bowl, mix pudding with milk, peppermint extract, and food coloring. Stir constantly with a wire whisk for 2 minutes. Refrigerate for 5 minutes.

Add whipped topping and mix well. Spoon the pudding mixture in a medium serving bowl or individual parfait glasses.

Top with crushed chocolate graham crackers.

Lemon Parfait

1 small box (0.3 ounces) sugar-free lemon-flavored gelatin
3/4 cup boiling water
1/2 cup very cold water
ice cubes
1 1/2 cups fat-free whipped topping
orange slices for garnish (optional)

Dissolve gelatin in boiling water, stirring constantly for 2 minutes.

Mix 1/2 cup very cold water with ice cubes to make 1 1/4 cups. Add to gelatin, stirring until slightly thickened. Remove any remaining ice cubes. Add whipped topping and mix well with a wire whisk.

Refrigerate for 30 minutes for a soft set and 1 1/2 hours for a firm set. Serve in individual parfait glasses or in a large glass bowl. Garnish with orange slices.

VARIATION: *Layered Parfait*–Double or triple this recipe, using two or three different flavors of gelatin, each prepared separately. Layer each flavor in a large glass serving bowl or parfait glasses. This makes a colorful presentation.

You'll find this creamy dessert to be light and fluffy. The refreshing taste is a great ending to any meal. Any flavor of gelatin can be substituted for the lemon.

Makes 3 1/2 cups
4 servings

Each Serving
3/4 cup

Carb Servings
1/2

Exchanges
1/2 carbohydrate

Nutrient Analysis
calories 55
total fat 0g
saturated fat 0g
cholesterol 0mg
sodium 70mg
total carbohydrate 10g
dietary fiber 0g
sugars 3g
protein 1g

This light dessert tastes and looks so good. It is especially attractive if layered in parfait glasses.

Makes 8 servings
6 cups

Each Serving
3/4 cup

Carb Servings
2

Exchanges
2 carbohydrate

Nutrient Analysis
calories 142
total fat 2g
saturated fat 1g
cholesterol 8mg
sodium 269mg
total carbohydrate 26g
dietary fiber 1g
sugars 18g
protein 3g

Cherry Cream Cheese Dessert

1 small box (1 ounce) sugar-free instant cheesecake pudding
2 cups fat-free milk
4 ounces light cream cheese (room temperature)
2 cups fat-free whipped topping
1 can (20 ounces) light cherry filling

In a small mixing bowl, combine pudding mix and milk. Beat on low speed to mix ingredients. Add cream cheese. Increase speed and beat until smooth and thickened. Refrigerate for 5 minutes.

Add whipped topping and mix well. Pour into individual parfait dishes or a large serving dish.

Top with pie filling.

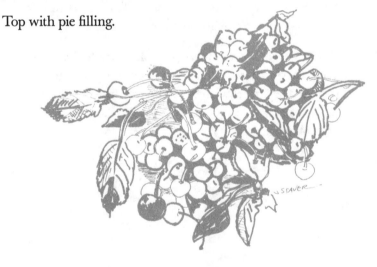

Fruit Pizza for a Crowd

1 package (18 ounces) sugar cookie dough
1 small box (1 ounce) sugar-free instant cheesecake
   pudding
2 cups fat-free milk
2 cups fat-free whipped topping
1 quart strawberries, washed and hulled (or other
   fresh fruit)

Preheat oven to 350 degrees. Spray a 16-inch pizza pan
with nonstick cooking spray.

Slice cookie dough into 1/4-inch thick slices. Arrange slices
on pizza pan so that they are 1/2 to 1 inch apart. Bake for
18–20 minutes or until golden and set. Cool.

In a medium bowl, mix pudding with milk. Stir
constantly with a wire whisk for 2 minutes. Refrigerate for
5 minutes.

Add whipped topping and mix well. Spread over cooled
cookie crust. Arrange fruit on top.

NOTE: This recipe will also make four 8-inch pizzas or
     one 11-inch by 14-inch and an 8-inch pizza. 8-
     inch cake pans work fine.

VARIATION: *Fruit Pizza Cookies*–Bake 18 individual
cookies, according to package directions. Cool. Top with
3 tablespoons of prepared pudding/whipped topping
mixture. Top with fresh fruit.

*I get lots of compliments
when I make this because
it looks so impressive. The
secret is arranging the fruit
in an attractive pattern. I
often use a combination of
strawberries, raspberries,
blueberries, and kiwi fruit.*

Makes 18 servings

Each Serving

Carb Servings
1 1/2

Exchanges
1 1/2 carbohydrate
1 fat

Nutrient Analysis
calories 155
total fat 5g
saturated fat 1g
cholesterol 55mg
sodium 254mg
total carbohydrate 25g
dietary fiber 1g
sugars 13g
protein 3g

Strawberry lovers will enjoy this refreshing dessert. The rich taste of the sour cream and the lightness of the whipped topping make this especially enjoyable.

Makes 4 cups
4 servings

Each Serving
1 cup

Carb Servings
1 1/2

Exchanges
1/2 carbohydrate
1 fruit

Nutrient Analysis
calories 106
total fat 1g
saturated fat 0g
cholesterol 0mg
sodium 58mg
total carbohydrate 23g
dietary fiber 3g
sugars 13g
protein 3g

Strawberries Romanoff

1/2 cup fat-free sour cream
1 tablespoon fat-free milk
1 cup fat-free whipped topping
4 cups strawberries, sliced
sugar or artificial sweetener to sweeten strawberries (optional)
4 whole strawberries for garnish

In a small bowl, mix sour cream with milk. Using a wire whisk, mix in whipped topping.

Sweeten strawberries, if needed.

Just before serving, layer in individual parfait glasses or in a medium-size glass bowl. Layer in this order: half of the strawberries, half of the sour cream mixture, half of the strawberries, and the remainder of the sour cream mixture.

Garnish with a whole strawberry.

NOTE: One serving is a good source of fiber.

VARIATION: *Peaches Romanoff*—substitute fresh peaches for the strawberries.

Cream Cheese Topping

1 small box (1 ounce) sugar-free instant cheesecake or
  vanilla pudding
2 cups fat-free milk
6 ounces fat-free cream cheese (room temperature)

In a small mixing bowl, combine pudding mix and milk.
Beat on low speed to mix well.

Add cream cheese. Increase speed and beat until smooth
and thick.

*Use as frosting in place
of traditional high-fat
cream cheese frosting.*

Makes 2 1/2 cups
20 servings

Each Serving
2 tablespoons

Carb Servings
0

Exchanges
free

Nutrient Analysis
calories 21
total fat 0g
saturated fat 0g
cholesterol 0mg
sodium 126mg
total carbohydrate 3g
dietary fiber 0g
sugars 2g
protein 2g

This is a fat-free version of a smoothie. You can eat it with a spoon or increase the milk and make a beverage.

Makes 1 serving

Each Serving

Carb Servings
1

Exchanges
1/2 fruit
1/2 fat-free milk

Nutrient Analysis
calories 91—with artificial sweetener 74
total fat 0g
saturated fat 0g
cholesterol 2mg
sodium 51mg
total carbohydrate 17g—with artificial sweetener 13g
dietary fiber 4g
sugars 13g—with artificial sweetener 9g
protein 5g

Fruit Slush

1/2–3/4 cup frozen fruit
1/2 cup fat-free milk, buttermilk, or fat-free plain yogurt
1/4 teaspoon vanilla extract
sweetener as needed: about 1–2 teaspoons sugar or the equivalent in artificial sweetener

Blend the first three ingredients until smooth.

Sweeten to taste.

NOTE: One serving is a good source of fiber.

Apple Crisp

6 cups peeled, sliced apples
1/4 cup water
2 tablespoons firmly packed brown sugar or the
 equivalent in artificial sweetener
2 teaspoons lemon juice
1 teaspoon ground cinnamon
1/2 cup oats (old-fashioned or quick)
1 tablespoon firmly packed brown sugar or the equivalent
 in artificial sweetener
1 tablespoon soft margarine

Preheat oven to 375 degrees.

Combine the first five ingredients and mix well. Arrange
apple mixture in an 8-inch by 8-inch baking dish that has
been sprayed with nonstick cooking spray.

Combine remaining ingredients and sprinkle
over apples. Bake for 30 minutes or
until apples are tender.

This old-fashioned dessert is good served warm or cold. See page 4 for information on using artificial sweetener.

Makes 8 servings

Each Serving

Carb Servings
1

Exchanges
1 carbohydrate

Nutrient Analysis
calories 88—with artificial
 sweetener 68
total fat 1g
saturated fat 0g
cholesterol 0mg
sodium 16mg
total carbohydrate 19g—
 with artificial sweetener
 14g
dietary fiber 2g
sugars 13g—with artificial
 sweetener 8g
protein 1g

Apple Cake

Makes 16 servings

Each Serving

Carb Servings
1 1/2—with artificial sweetener 1
1/2 fat

Exchanges
1 1/2 carbohydrate—with artificial sweetener 1
1/2 fat

Nutrient Analysis
calories 142—with artificial sweetener 110
total fat 4g
saturated fat 0g
cholesterol 0mg
sodium 135mg
total carbohydrate 25g—with artificial sweetener 17g
dietary fiber 2g
sugars 15g—with artificial sweetener 7g
protein 2g

2/3 cup granulated sugar or the equivalent in artificial sweetener
1/2 cup brown sugar
1/2 cup egg substitute (equal to 2 eggs)
1/4 cup canola oil
2/3 cup unbleached all-purpose flour
2/3 cup whole-wheat flour
1/2 cup oat bran
1 1/2 teaspoons baking soda
1 teaspoon ground cinnamon
1/4 teaspoon ground allspice
3 cups finely chopped apples (unpeeled)

Optional topping
3/4 cup oats (quick or old fashioned)
1 1/2 tablespoons firmly packed brown sugar
1 1/2 tablespoons soft margarine

Preheat oven to 350 degrees. In a small bowl, mix sugars, egg, and oil until well blended.

Mix remaining ingredients, except apples, in a large bowl.

Add egg mixture to dry ingredients and mix just until moistened. Stir in apples. Pour into a 9-inch by 13-inch baking pan that has been sprayed with nonstick cooking spray. If using optional topping, combine the ingredients and sprinkle over cake batter. Bake for 25–30 minutes.

Butterfly Cupcakes

1 small box (1 ounce) sugar-free instant vanilla
   pudding mix
2 cups fat-free milk
1 dozen cupcakes, yellow or white
2 tablespoons sugar-free preserves (raspberry or
   strawberry)
powdered sugar (optional)

Make pudding according to package directions, using fat-free milk. Let set in refrigerator for 5 minutes.

Cut a cone shape from the top
of each cupcake, according to
diagram, and set aside.

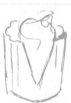

Fill cavity of each
cupcake with 1 tablespoon
of pudding.

Cut cones in half to
make wings.

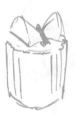

Place two halves, flat side down,
on each cupcake to represent
butterfly wings.

Place 1/2 teaspoon of preserves in the
center to resemble the body. Dust with
powdered sugar (optional).

VARIATION: *Chocolate Butterfly Cupcakes*—Substitute
chocolate cupcakes and fill with fat-free whipped topping.

*My mother used to make
these for school parties
when I was a child. They
are so special because each
cupcake looks like it has a
butterfly sitting on its top.*

Makes 12 servings
(plus extra pudding)

Each Serving
1 cupcake

Carb Servings
1 1/2

Exchanges
1 1/2 carbohydrate
1/2 fat

Nutrient Analysis
calories 140
total fat 4g
saturated fat 1g
cholesterol 11mg
sodium 273mg
total carbohydrate 23g
dietary fiber 1g
sugars 3g
protein 3g

Makes 9 servings

Each Serving

Carb Servings
1 1/2—with artificial sweetener 1

Exchanges
1 1/2 carbohydrate—with artificial sweetener 1
1/2 fat

Nutrient Analysis
calories 134—with artificial sweetener 112
total fat 3g
saturated fat 0g
cholesterol 0mg
sodium 154mg
total carbohydrate 24g—with artificial sweetener 18g
dietary fiber 1g
sugars 13g—with artificial sweetener 8g
protein 2g

Mandarin Orange Cake

1 cup unbleached all-purpose flour
1/2 cup granulated sugar, or 1/4 cup of sugar and the equivalent in artificial sweetener for 1/4 cup sugar
1 teaspoon baking soda
1/2 teaspoon salt (optional)
1 can (11 ounces) mandarin oranges, in juice, drained
1/4 cup egg substitute (equal to 1 egg)
2 tablespoons canola oil
1 teaspoon vanilla extract

Preheat oven to 350 degrees. Mix the first four ingredients in a medium bowl.

Combine the remaining ingredients, mashing the oranges. Combine with the dry ingredients and mix well.

Pour into an 8-inch by 8-inch baking pan that has been sprayed with nonstick cooking spray. Bake for 30–35 minutes.

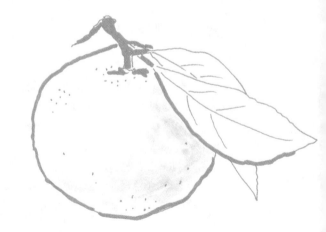

Pineapple Cake

2 cups unbleached all-purpose flour

1 cup granulated sugar, or 1/2 cup sugar and the equivalent in artificial sweetener for 1/2 cup sugar

2 teaspoons baking soda

1/4 teaspoon salt (optional)

1 can (20 ounces) unsweetened crushed pineapple, in juice (not drained)

1/2 cup egg substitute (equal to 2 eggs)

Preheat oven to 350 degrees. Combine the first four ingredients in a medium bowl.

Mix pineapple with egg substitute. Add to dry ingredients and mix until blended.

Pour into a 9-inch by 13-inch baking pan that has been sprayed with nonstick cooking spray. Bake for 30–35 minutes.

This moist cake does not use any fat. It can be served plain, or with fat-free whipped topping. Cream Cheese Topping is also good on this cake. See page 4 for information on using artificial sweetener.

Makes 16 servings

Each Serving

Carb Servings
2—with artificial sweetener 1 1/2

Exchanges
2 carbohydrate—with artificial sweetener 1 1/2

Nutrient Analysis
calories 121—with artificial sweetener 96
total fat 0g
saturated fat 0g
cholesterol 0mg
sodium 172mg
total carbohydrate 28g—with artificial sweetener 21g
dietary fiber 1g
sugars 15g—with artificial sweetener 9g
protein 3g

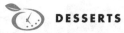

Index

Other Books from Small Steps Press

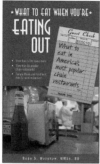

What To Eat When You're Eating Out
by Hope S. Warshaw, MMSc, RD, CDE, BC-ADM
Eat out without guilt or sacrifice! This bestselling guide features more than 5,000 menu items for over 60 restaurant chains. This is the most comprehensive guide to restaurant nutrition for people who like to eat out.
Order no. 4723-01; Price $9.95

The Ultimate Calorie, Carb, & Fat Gram Counter
by Lea Ann Holzmeister, RD, CDE
Registered dietitian Lea Ann Holzmeister has put together complete nutritional information, including carbs, fat, calories, and more for nearly 7,000 listings, as well as charts for fast foods and prepackaged meals.
Order no. 4724-01; Price $9.95

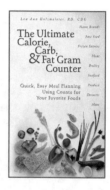

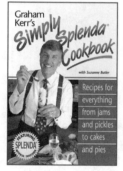

Graham Kerr's Simply Splenda® Cookbook
by Graham Kerr, with Suzanne Butler
Graham Kerr and his wife, Treena, have made it their crusade to help others learn to cook wisely and to live well, proving that with wise food choices, it is possible to be well even after the diagnosis of a chronic disease. Includes 75 delicious recipes, made with better nutrition, fewer carbohydrates, and great taste!
Order no. 4649-01; Price $12.95

The Healthy Lunchbox
by Marie McClendon and Cristy Shauck
The Healthy Lunchbox is filled with tips, tricks, and techniques for organizing and preparing quick and easy meals with a little more zing–and a lot more nutrition– than those boring old sandwiches, chips, and sodas.
Order no. 5013-01; Price $12.95

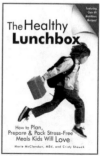

To order these and other great Small Steps Press titles, call **1-800-232-6733** or visit ***www.smallstepspress.com***. Small Steps Press titles are also available in bookstores nationwide.

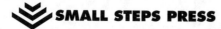